Gluten-Free Holiday Baking

More than 150 Cakes, Pies, and Pastries Made with Flavor, Not Flour

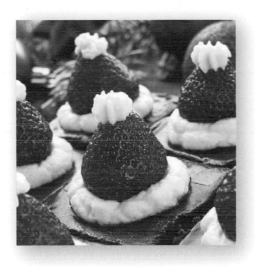

Ellen Brown

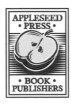

APPLESEED
· PRESS ·

· BOOK ·
PUBLISHERS

Kennebunkport, Maine

Design by Alicia Freile, Tango Media
Typeset by Gwen Galeone, Tango Media
Typography: Chaparral Pro, Helvetica Neue, and Latino Rumba

Photos Copyright: page 5, M. Unal Ozmen; page 7, Picsfive; page 8, marco mayer, nastiakru, Francesco83, Hana Sichyngrová, Robyn Mackenzie, Marie C Fields; page 9, marekuliasz; page 15 (top), David P. Smith; page 15 (bottom), Coprid; page 19, hd connelly; page 23, sarsmis; page 24, Mark Stout Photography; page 27, Elena Elisseeva; page 28, Letterberry; page 31, Nataliya Peregudova; page 32, Letterberry; page 35, pearl7; page 36, Foodpictures; page 39, Marcel Jancovic; page 40, Feng Yu; page 43, margouillat photo; page 44, AGfoto; page 47, AGfoto; page 48, TigerForce; page 51, AGfoto; page 52, Donatella Tandelli; page 57, Gayvoronskaya_Yana; page 58, Mariya Volik; page 61, Simone van den Berg; page 62, Lilya; page 65, HG Photography; page 66, 54613; page 69, Shebeko; page 70, Lilyana Vynogradova; page 73, sarsmis; page 74, Daniel Korzeniewski; page 77, 29september; page 78, jreika; page 82, biburcha; page 85, SCPixBit (S. Chiariello); page 86, AGfoto; page 89, hd connelly; page 90, Adrian Britton; page 93, George Bailey; page 94, Luiz Rocha; page 97, Laura Adamache; page 98, Darren K. Fisher; page 101, tremble; page 102, Jesse Kunerth; page 105, Liz Van Steenburgh; page 106, Sharon Day; page 109, Marie C Fields; page 110, Steman Shots; page 115, Joe Gough; page 116, Mykhaylo Feshchur; page 119, msheldrake; page 120, Komar Maria; page 123, joanna wnuk; page 124, HLPhoto; page 127, Againstar; page 128, Jump Photography; page 131, Solaria; page 132, rawcaptured; page 135, julesclancy; page 136, Viktor1; page 139, Christopher Halloran; page 140, Wiktory. All used under license from Shutterstock.com

Manufactured in China

2 4 6 8 10 9 7 5 3 1

The publisher makes no warranties and accepts no liability or responsibility for any health problems, consequences, or symptoms that arise from eating the foods presented within this book. Several ingredients throughout this book are known food allergens. One should consult a doctor or health care provider to determine if one has food allergies or any other medical condition(s) that would conflict with the ingredients included within this work.

Contents

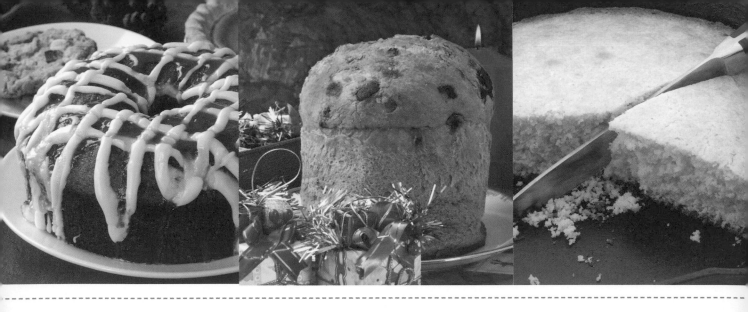

Introduction

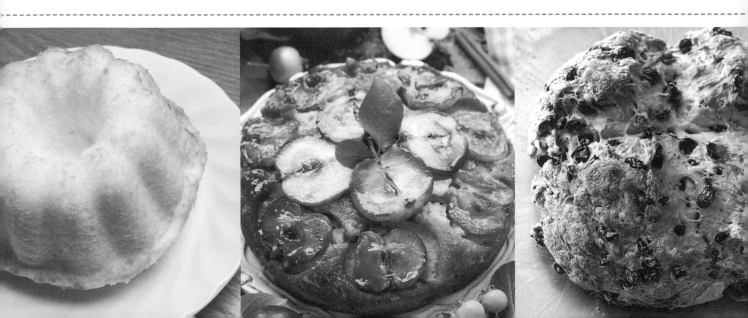

It's not easy to follow a gluten-free diet, especially around the holidays. We all want "visions of sugarplums." I'm here to tell you that it is possible to have them when you make baked goods yourself at home.

Understanding the need to live gluten-free starts with understanding how gluten can cause life-threatening problems if not removed from the diet of those who cannot tolerate it. But the good news is that following a gluten-free diet can mitigate debilitating symptoms and pain in as little as a few months—using food rather than a pharmacy. Those following a gluten-free diet need not be deprived of baked goods as delicious as those made with gluten— from rich cakes to crispy breads and gooey pies.

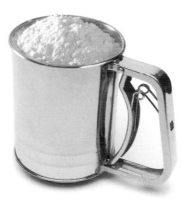

Our bodies contain a complex and interlocking system to prevent harm. There is a network of organs, glands, and cell types all dedicated to warding off illness lumped under the heading of the immune system. But sometimes the immune system attacks healthy cells rather than potentially harmful ones. These maladies are termed *autoimmune diseases*.

Autoimmune disorders are not fully understood, but many medical authorities now accept some causes. The sources of these disorders include viruses that change the information carried inside the cells, sunlight and other forms of radiation, certain chemicals, and pharmaceuticals. There is also believed to be a connection to sex hormones; many more women than men suffer from autoimmune disorders.

There are more than eighty types of autoimmune disease, and they include lupus, rheumatoid arthritis, and Graves' disease. Some medical authorities also believe that multiple sclerosis is caused by an autoimmune response. While the aggravating factors in many of these diseases are complex, in the case of celiac disease it is really rather easy. Celiac disease is caused by an autoimmune response to gluten, one of the thirty proteins found in wheat, barley, and rye.

Humans as a species are unable to properly digest the gluten protein. Normal protein digestion involves a complete breakdown of protein into small particles called amino acids that are in turn absorbed by the small intestine and used by the body as a nutritional source. Many people appear unaffected by being unable to digest gluten properly.

But for those who are intolerant, the undigested gluten protein gets absorbed into the lining of the small intestine but is not seen by the body as a source of nutrition. The body's immune system attacks these protein particles as something that needs to be destroyed, in very much the same way as it would attack an invading organism such as a virus, bacterium, or parasite. The attack by the immune system causes inflammation and damage to the small intestine, which prevents it from absorbing the nutrients from food that are important for staying healthy.

Normally, the small intestine is lined with tiny, hair-like projections called *villi* that resemble the deep pile of a plush carpet on a microscopic scale. It is these villi that work to absorb vitamins, minerals, and other nutrients from the food you eat. Without prominent *villi*, the inner surface of the small intestine becomes less like a plush carpet and more like a tile floor. The body is unable to absorb nutrients necessary for health and growth, resulting in malnutrition.

It is now clear that the disease is far more common than doctors once believed. New research reveals that celiac disease may be one of the most common genetic diseases, and one federal study estimates that 1 in every 133 Americans suffers from celiac disease; that's more than 3 million people.

The condition is diagnosed by testing for three antibodies—anti-gliadin, anti-endomysial, and anti-tissue transglutaminase—all of which are present when an affected person is exposed to gluten but disappear when the offending grains are no longer consumed.

But there are millions more people whose digestive problems don't fall under the strict definition of celiac disease because they do not test positively for the antibodies but who have found that following a gluten-free diet helps them. Rather than terming them *gluten-intolerant,* they're termed *gluten-sensitive,* and this group could include up to 30 percent of the American population.

For this much larger group, eliminating gluten can eliminate symptoms ranging from abdominal pain to osteoporosis and sinus congestion. Gluten-sensitivity has also been linked to conditions such as psoriasis, anemia, and asthma.

Following a gluten-free diet is not a temporary measure to ameliorate a condition. It's for life. Eliminating gluten doesn't cause the body to become less sensitive to it. The condition for which the gluten was eliminated can return as soon as gluten is reintroduced to the diet.

Avoiding Contamination

If you're new to gluten-free baking, or you're making these treats as a gift for someone who must follow a gluten-free diet, the whole concept of contamination is perhaps new to you as well. Setting up your system so that gluten-free foods and foods containing gluten never meet can take time, but it is time well spent.

Here are some rules to follow to ensure that your gluten-free products are not inadvertently contaminated by wheat flour or any gluten-containing food:

• Thoroughly wash cabinets where gluten-free products will be stored, and be sure everyone who uses the kitchen is aware that these cabinets contain only gluten-free food. Even so, unless the kitchen is to be free of all gluten-containing foods, it's still wise to place gluten-free ingredients in airtight containers before storing them.
• Clean all the kitchen surfaces thoroughly before starting to prepare gluten-free dishes, and then change the dishrag and dishtowel for a fresh one. Don't use a sponge because it cannot be properly cleaned to make it free from gluten. The same is true for porous surfaces such as wooden cutting boards. Have special ones for gluten-free ingredients.

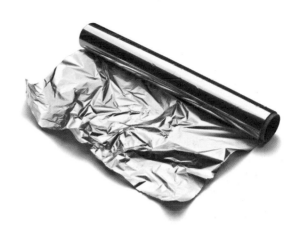

Foil is useful for keeping foods separate.

• Have separate containers of butter or margarine for gluten-free baking. Crumbs from someone's morning toast could have landed on a stick of butter at breakfast.
• Don't use the same sifter for gluten-free and regular flours. Label the gluten-free sifter to avoid mistakes.
• Have separate containers of ingredients for all gluten-free baking. Even though there is no gluten in granulated sugar or baking soda, molecules of wheat flour could have landed on them.
• Always place the gluten-free foods on the top shelf of the oven to avoid the risk of spills onto it. The same is true in the refrigerator; the gluten-free foods should be on higher shelves.
• Foil is a great way to avoid contamination. Use foil to keep foods separate when preparing, cooking, or storing.
• Use stickers of different colors when storing gluten-free foods to segregate them from other foods.

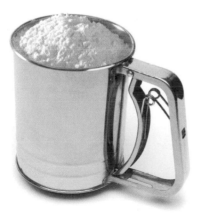

Label a gluten-free sifter so that it doesn't get used with wheat flour.

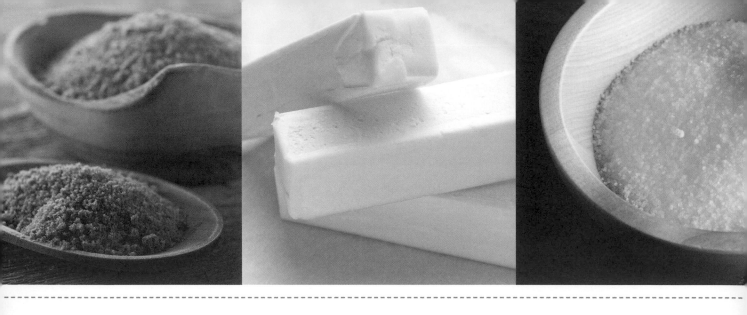

CHAPTER 1:

The Gluten-Free Pantry and Baking Basics

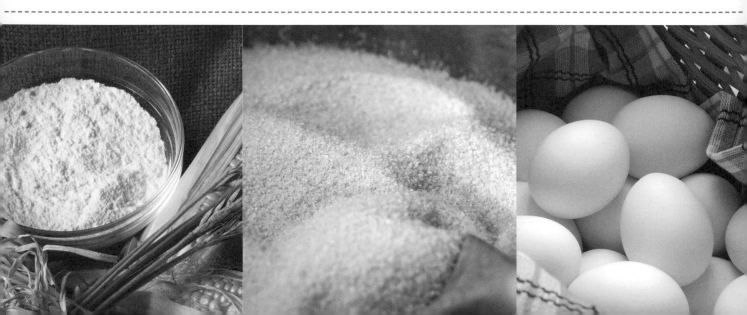

M ost of the ingredients used to make the delicious treats in this book are very familiar. They've been part of every cook's repertoire since that first venture into the kitchen to make a batch of brownies as a child. Listed in the ingredients are old friends such as eggs, butter, baking soda, and vanilla.

The dough or batter can be flavored with chocolate in many forms, as well as by adding citrus and other fruits. Some recipes contain crunchy nuts, while others have succulent dried fruits folded in.

One ingredient crucial to traditional baking is not listed—all-purpose flour. And that omission creates a sea change. There is no one powdery substance that can take the place of wheat flour and the gluten produced by two of its inherent proteins.

Gluten is a beautiful thing. Who doesn't love a crusty bread or a tender and moist cake? Traditionally, gluten has been the way to achieve this range of textures.

To make gluten-free baked goods just as tantalizing as ones made with wheat flour requires more than one dry ingredient and a slightly different proportion of dry and wet components. In this chapter you will learn about these all-natural foods and the role they play in creating baked goods that will bring a sparkle to everyone's eyes as bright as the lights on the Christmas tree.

The Role of Gluten in Traditional Baking

Although there's some science involved with all cooking, when the end result is a baked good, science and art are given almost equal billing, with science leading the way. Eliminating rye and barley from the diet presents some challenges, but eliminating all forms of wheat and wheat flour is a Herculean task—especially especially baking. For centuries, wheat flour has been a key ingredient in most recipes.

Wheat flour contains as many as thirty proteins, and two of those—glutenin and gliadin—form gluten when stirred with moisture. These two proteins grab water and connect to form elastic strands of gluten. If flour has a lot of these proteins, it grabs up water faster, making the strong and springy gluten that is needed to bake bread. If there are fewer proteins or if the proteins are coated with fat to become shorter, the gluten creates tenderness as in piecrust.

The formation of this elastic gluten network serves many functions in a recipe. Like a net, gluten traps and holds air bubbles. They later expand from the gas created by leavening agent like baking soda or baking powder. When a recipe is baked, the stretched flour proteins become rigid as moisture evaporates from the heat of the oven, and sets the baked goods' structure.

Replicating this structure is no easy task. There is no magic wand to wave that can remove the gluten from wheat flour because the proteins are built into the DNA of the wheat plant. But with a adding a few other dry powders, the results can be just as good.

> When you're watching out for wheat by reading ingredient labels, there are other ways it can be listed. Both kamut and faro are ancient types of wheat, and bulgur is cracked wheat kernels. Also be on the lookout for couscous, which is a granular pasta made with wheat flour. Other ways wheat flour is listed include semolina, farina, and durum.

Gluten-Free Flours and Starches

Here's the bad news: There is no one ingredient with which you can make a one-to-one substitution for all-purpose wheat flour when making gluten-free baked goods. But here's the good news: Although the recipes might appear long because you need several ingredients to create the same texture imparted by using wheat flour, the ingredients are readily available even in general supermarkets.

If you visit the gluten-free baking aisle of supermarkets or go to websites you'll discover there is a dizzying array of products that can be used to replace wheat flour. In addition to being free of gluten, many of these ingredients are far more nutritious than wheat flour.

Each substance in the gluten-free arsenal has different properties. One will strengthen, another will act as a tenderizer, and another will add moisture. Wheat has all of these properties, so it is not difficult to understand needing multiple flours to substitute for just one.

There are two basic categories of ingredients:
- **Protein/fiber flours,** such as white and brown rice flour, provide structure, stability, flavor, color, texture, and nutrition. Some flours in this category, such as bean flour and chestnut flour, add flavor as well as texture, so they are not used very often. But they should be used for gluten-free general cooking.
- **Starches,** such as cornstarch, tapioca starch, potato starch, and sweet rice flour, are very fine in texture and create baked goods that have a soft crumb and a smooth texture.

Protein/fiber flours are heavy and baked goods end up very dense. Starches alone cannot provide enough structure for baked goods to hold their shape. Successful gluten-free baking begins with using the right flour blend—using *both* protein/fiber flours and starches together to get good results. The right combination can produce excellent results, often indistinguishable from baked goods made with wheat.

Flours should be stored refrigerated after opening; starches can be stored at room temperature. If you have pre-mixed a baking mix, it's best to store it refrigerated if you have space.

The ingredients listed here are the ones used in this book. There are many other ones out there, but I tried to keep the list basic rather than have you go to the expense of buying myriad products.

Almond meal: Of the nut flours, this is the only one that is available prepackaged because it has been used for centuries for so many desserts, such as classic French macaroons. You can grind blanched almonds in a coffee grinder or mini-food processor to make your own. You can also substitute nuts such as peeled hazelnuts for almonds.

Amaranth flour: Amaranth is a tiny seed native to Central America; it was one of the primary grains raised by the Aztecs. The flour is much higher in lysine, an essential amino acid, than other grain flours. When amaranth is combined with cornmeal it creates a complete protein like that found in meat or poultry.

Arrowroot: This starchy flour, made by drying and grinding the roots of a tropical tuber, has twice the thickening power of wheat flour and is completely tasteless. It is most often used to thicken sauces and puddings but can also be used in baked goods. It can be substituted on a one-to-one basis for cornstarch.

Cornmeal: We are all familiar with cornmeal, and it is important to buy one from a manufacturer who processes it in a facility not contaminated with gluten. Cornmeal is made by grinding dried corn kernels. Cornmeal can be fine-, medium-, or coarse-textured. Water-ground or stone-ground types are more nutritious than steel-ground, since more of the corn kernel is retained.

Cornstarch: Along with arrowroot, cornstarch is what is most often used to thicken gluten-free foods as well as in baking. Called *corn flour* in some countries, it should never be confused with cornmeal. Cornstarch is made by grinding the endosperm of the corn kernel after the kernels have been steeped for a few days, which makes it possible to separate the germ from the endosperm.

Potato starch: Potato starch is very different from potato flour, so be careful when you shop for it. Potato starch is made from raw potatoes, while potato flour is made from cooked potatoes. The flour is far denser, and the two cannot be substituted for each other.

Rice flour: This neutral-flavored flour is one of the most common substitutes for all-purpose wheat flour. Both white and brown rice can be made into flour, but the outer husk is always removed before grinding. Brown rice flour has a better nutritional profile because it does contain some fiber. I use both in these recipes, and the choice really depends on the desired color of the baked cookie.

Sweet rice flour: Called *mochiko* in Japanese, it can be found in Asian markets as well as supermarkets, and though it is called *sweet* there is no sweetening added. It's made from glutinous short-grained Japanese rice, and it makes cookie dough pliable and somewhat sticky. If you are out of sweet rice flour, the closest substitution is tapioca starch.

Tapioca flour: Also called *cassava flour*, tapica flour derived from the yucca plant, which is a starchy tropical tuber. It adds body to baked goods as well as a chewy texture, and it helps baked goods to brown.

> Oats do not contain gluten, but the problem is possible contamination of oats with gluten-containing grains grown nearby. Pure oats—those not contaminated by other grains—are recommended by a majority of celiac organizations in North America, and should say *gluten-free* or *non-contaminated* on the package.

Gums as Binders

Gluten gives doughs and batters strength so that the air incorporated by yeast or chemical leavening agents is trapped until the heat of the oven cooks the proteins and forms a structure. Your cakes or pie crusts might end up as a pile of crumbs if it were not for the additions of natural gums to serve as binders and give gluten-free flours and starches that all-important "stretch factor." They also give doughs and batters the inherent stickiness we recognize.

The two different powdered products that can be used interchangeably are xanthan (pronounced ZAHN-*thun*) gum and guar (pronounced *gwar*) gum. They are mixed with the dry ingredients and added along with them to the mixture.

Xanthan gum. Sometimes called *corn sugar gum,* it's a natural carbohydrate that isn't absorbed by the body. The additive is produced by the fermentation of the bacteria *Xanthomonas campestris*. When this bacterium is combined with corn sugar, it creates a colorless slime, which is then dehydrated and ground into xanthan gum.

Guar gum. The guar plant, also known as a cluster plant, grows primarily in areas of Pakistan and the northern parts of India that share a climate of alternating monsoons and droughts. In these regions it represents an important crop. The plants are harvested after the monsoon season and the seeds are allowed to dry in the sun. The seeds are then manually or mechanically separated and processed into powder or sold as split seeds.

> You've eaten xanthan gum many times, and if you see it on a label it's a real food and not something out of a test tube. Manufacturers add xanthan gum to candy to prevent sugar crystals from forming and to many ice creams to give them a smooth texture.

Basic Baking Mixture and Recipe Conversion

What percentage of which flour and starch to use depends on the type of baked good you're making. When baking with wheat flour there is a wide range available depending on the use. For example, bread flour is very high in protein from its base of hard wheat; cake flour is very low in protein and is comprised of soft wheat; all-purpose flour blends the two.

There are a few all-purpose gluten-free baking blends on the market, but I think the same strategy of designing a mix to the type of baked good is preferable. This formulation is one I devised that works for many recipes, and it can be used once blended in a one-to-one substitution for all-purpose wheat flour. Use this formulation when converting family favorites for gluten-free baking, but use the precise formulation given with the recipes in this book for these dishes. I've developed them carefully to maximize the flavor and texture of each dish.

It is based on rice flour with a few starches plus xanthan gum. You can substitute up to 1 cup of almond meal for 1 cup of the rice flour for nut cookies.

Basic Baking Mix

Makes 3 cups

2 cups white or brown rice flour
⅓ cup sweet rice flour
⅓ cup potato starch
⅓ cup tapioca starch
2 teaspoons xanthan gum

Mix all ingredients together, and store refrigerated in an airtight container.

Other Helpful Ingredients

Although gluten-free baking presents some unique challenges, other than the choice of dry ingredients the recipes follow centuries of traditions in combinations of ingredients that work well together.

Eggs: Without the protein being supplied by the gluten in the flour, eggs take on a more important role; they are another great source of protein and can create the structure of baked goods. In addition to providing protein, they also create the steam needed for starches to become firm. Egg yolk is also a rich source of emulsifying agents that makes it easier to incorporate air into the doughs and batters due to its fat and lecithin content.

Sugar: Sugar adds sweetness, as well as contributing to the browning process that takes place when a baked good is cooked. The browning occurs when the sugar reacts with the protein in eggs and the dairy solids of butter during baking, and the higher the sugar content of cookie dough, the browner it will become once baked. Sugar also holds moisture, which extends the life of baked goods. Along with solid fat, it is the crystals of sugar that makes small holes, which are expanded by leavening agents.

> The granulated sugar we take for granted today as a staple was once so rare and expensive it was called "white gold." Sugar cane, the first source of sugar, is a perennial grass that originated in Asia but is now grown in virtually every tropical and subtropical region of the world. It was only during the nineteenth century that refining beets for their sugar became commonplace.

Fats: In all baking, where solid fats are creamed with crystalline sugar, tiny air cells are incorporated into the batter so the baked good will have a fine, aerated texture. Fat is also responsible for providing lubrication and a luxurious mouth feel. I am a devotee of baking with only unsalted butter. The milk fat in butter contributes tenderness, color, and helps build the structure of baked good. But most importantly, it releases its delicious flavor.

Leavening agents: A leavening agent is anything that creates volume in baked goods by foaming. Air is a natural leavener, which is why so many cake batters specify to beat the butter and sugar until that wonderful state of "light and fluffy." The lightness and the fluffiness is the air that's incorporated.

Most of the time the leavening is left to two primary chemical agents—**baking soda** and **baking powder**. Both of these produce carbon dioxide when they are mixed with moisture. Baking soda, also called *bicarbonate of soda,* must be combined with an acidic ingredient such as buttermilk to create carbon dioxide, while baking powder is a combination of baking soda and cream of tartar, which is acidic. Baking soda is twice as strong as baking powder, but the two can be substituted for one another.

It is important to look at baking powder carefully. Some brands use a small percentage of wheat starch as the "moisture absorption agent." Most, however, use cornstarch or potato starch, including such leading brands as Rumford and Davis, but do check labels carefully.

Baking Basics

Cooking is a form of art, but when it comes to baking science is also part of the equation. While savory recipes are tolerant of virtually endless substitutions, baked goods are not. Each ingredient performs a specific function in a recipe based on a certain quantity to create a batter or dough.

These are general pointers on procedures to be used for all genres of baked goods:

• **Measure accurately.** Measure dry ingredients in dry measuring cups, which are plastic or metal, and come in sizes of ¼, ⅓, ½, and 1 cup. Spoon dry ingredients from the container or canister into the measuring cup, and then sweep the top with a straight edge such as the back of a knife or a spatula to measure it properly. Do not dip the cup into the canister or tap it on the counter to produce a level surface. These methods pack down the dry ingredients and can increase the actual volume by up to 10 percent. Tablespoons and teaspoons should also be leveled; a rounded ½ teaspoon can really measure almost 1 teaspoon. If the box or can does not have a straight edge built in, level the excess in the spoon back into the container with the back of a knife blade. Measure liquids in liquid measures, which come in different sizes but are transparent glass or plastic and have lines on the sides. To accurately measure liquids, place the measuring cup on a flat counter and bend down to read the marked level.
• **Create consistent temperature.** All ingredients should be at room temperature unless otherwise indicated. Having all ingredients at the same temperature makes it easier to combine them into a smooth, homogeneous mixture. Adding cold liquid to a dough or batter can cause the batter to lose its unified structure by making the fat rigid.
• **Preheat the oven.** Some ovens can take up to 25 minutes to reach a high temperature such as 450°F. The minimum heating time should be 15 minutes.
• **Plan ahead.** Read the recipe thoroughly and assemble all your ingredients. Account for all ingredients required for a recipe in advance, so you don't get to a step and realize you must improvise. Assembling in advance also lessens the risk of over-mixing dough or batters as the mixer drones on while you search for a specific spice or bag of chips.

Careful Creaming

Perhaps the most vital step in the creation of a cake batter is the "creaming" of the butter and sugar. During this process air is beaten in and is trapped in the butter's crystalline structure. It is the number and size of the air bubbles (which then become enlarged by the carbon dioxide produced by baking soda or baking powder) that leavens a dough or batter to produce a high, finely-textured product.

The starting point in proper creaming is to ensure that the butter is at the correct temperature, approximately 70°F. Remove butter from the refrigerator and cut each stick into approximately 30 slices. Allow them to sit at room temperature for 15–20 minutes to soften.

Begin creaming by beating the butter alone in a mixer until it has broken into small pieces. Then add the sugar and beat at medium speed to start the process of combining them. Then increase the speed to high, and scrape the bowl frequently. When properly creamed, the texture of the butter and sugar mixture will be light and fluffy.

Important Equipment

There is very little specialized equipment needed for baking the recipes in this book. You'll need a selection of baking pans for the cakes and tortes in Chapter 2, a few pie plates, and some cookie sheets. Here is a list of the machines and gadgets I used on a regular basis developing the recipes for this book:

• **Microplane grater.** These resemble a flat kitchen spatula but with tiny holes in it. They're fabulous for grating citrus zest and fibrous foods such as ginger or nutmeg, and you can also use them for Parmesan cheese and even garlic cloves for other recipes.

• **Food processor.** There is a dedicated corner of my dishwasher given over to this workhorse of the kitchen. The base needs to be cleaned thoroughly before making any gluten-free item, but for very little money you can purchase a second work bowl. The work bowl of food processors is made of plastic that can harbor food particles once scratched.

• **Wire cooling racks.** Wire cooling racks are essential, and there's really no substitute for them. The type of rack on top of a broiler pan is too solid, and there's nothing that makes baked goods lose their texture—especially especially those made with gluten-free ingredients—faster than placing them on an impervious surface.

• **A powerful mixer.** Some of these bread doughs are very thick, and a standard mixer that sits on the counter is the best friend you can have. While hand-held mixers are fine for small tasks, the stand mixer is what is best for baking. The paddle attachment makes the thickest substance look easy to blend, and the dough hook takes all the labor out of kneading.

• **Offset spatulas.** An offset spatula is the type of spatula with the handle raised up from the level of the blade to make transferring cookies from the baking sheets to the cooling racks comfortable.

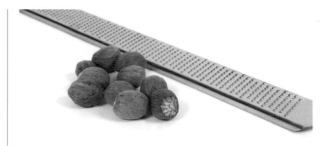

A microplane grater is excellent for grating nutmeg.

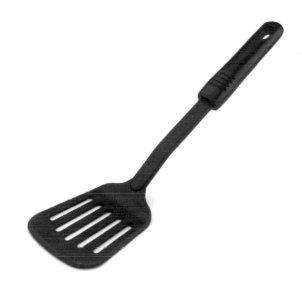

Using an offset spatula eases removes food from baking sheets.

Dressing Up Your Baked Goods

For the holidays you may want to add some extra treatment to baked goods. Here are some options consistent with a gluten-free diet.

Confectioners' Sugar Glaze

This is the easiest and most basic way to dress up a bread, muffin, or simple cake, and it hardens in less than an hour.

Yield: 1½ cups

Active time: 5 minutes

Start to finish: 5 minutes

4 cups (1 pound) confectioners' sugar

4–5 tablespoons water

½ teaspoon clear vanilla extract

Food coloring (optional)

1. Combine confectioners' sugar, 4 tablespoons water, and vanilla in a mixing bowl. Stir until smooth, adding additional water if too thick.

2. If tinting glaze, transfer it to small cups and add food coloring, a few drops at a time, until desired consistency is reached. Stir well before adding additional coloring.

Note: The glaze can be kept at room temperature in an airtight container, with a sheet of plastic wrap pressed directly into the surface, for up 6 hours. Beat it again lightly to emulsify before using.

Variations:
* *Substitute orange juice for the water and orange extract for the vanilla.*
* *Substitute peppermint oil or almond extract for the vanilla.*

Royal Icing

This is the formulation for the shiny icing used on many holiday breads and tortes. It should only be used, however, on baked goods that remain at room temperature because refrigeration can cause the frosting to become sticky.

Yield: 3½ cups

Active time: 5 minutes

Start to finish: 12 minutes

3 large egg whites, at room temperature

½ teaspoon cream of tartar

¼ teaspoon salt

4 cups (1 pound) confectioners' sugar

½ teaspoon pure vanilla extract

Food coloring (optional)

1. Place egg whites in a grease-free mixing bowl and beat at medium speed with an electric mixer until frothy. Add the cream of tartar and salt, raise the speed to high, and beat until soft peaks form.

2. Add sugar and beat at low speed to moisten. Raise the speed to high, and beat for 5–7 minutes, or until mixture is glossy and stiff peaks form. Beat in vanilla.

3. If tinting icing, transfer it to small cups and add food coloring, a few drops at a time, until desired consistency is reached. Stir well before adding additional coloring.

Note: The icing can be kept at room temperature in an airtight container for up to 2 days. Beat it again lightly to emulsify before using.

Variations:

✳ *Substitute peppermint oil, almond extract, lemon oil, or orange oil for the vanilla.*

Buttercream Icing

Buttercream Icing is richer than Royal Icing, and it is also not bright white because it's made with butter. It hardens somewhat but not into a true glaze. Buttercream is a wonderful icing to use to make rosettes or other complex decorations with a pastry bag; if the icing isn't stiff enough, add additional confectioners' sugar in 1-tablespoon increments.

Yield: 2½ cups

Active time: 5 minutes

Start to finish: 5 minutes

¼ pound (1 stick) unsalted butter, softened

4 cups (1 pound) confectioners' sugar

3 tablespoons milk

1 teaspoon pure vanilla extract

Food coloring (optional)

1. Place butter, sugar, milk, and vanilla in a large mixing bowl. Beat at low speed with an electric mixer to combine. Increase the speed to high, and beat for 2 minutes, or until light and fluffy.

2. If tinting icing, transfer it to small cups and add food coloring, a few drops at a time, until desired consistency is reached. Stir well before adding additional coloring.

Note: The icing can be kept refrigerated in an airtight container for up to 5 days. Bring it to room temperature before using.

Variations:
* *Substitute almond extract, lemon oil, or orange oil for the vanilla.*

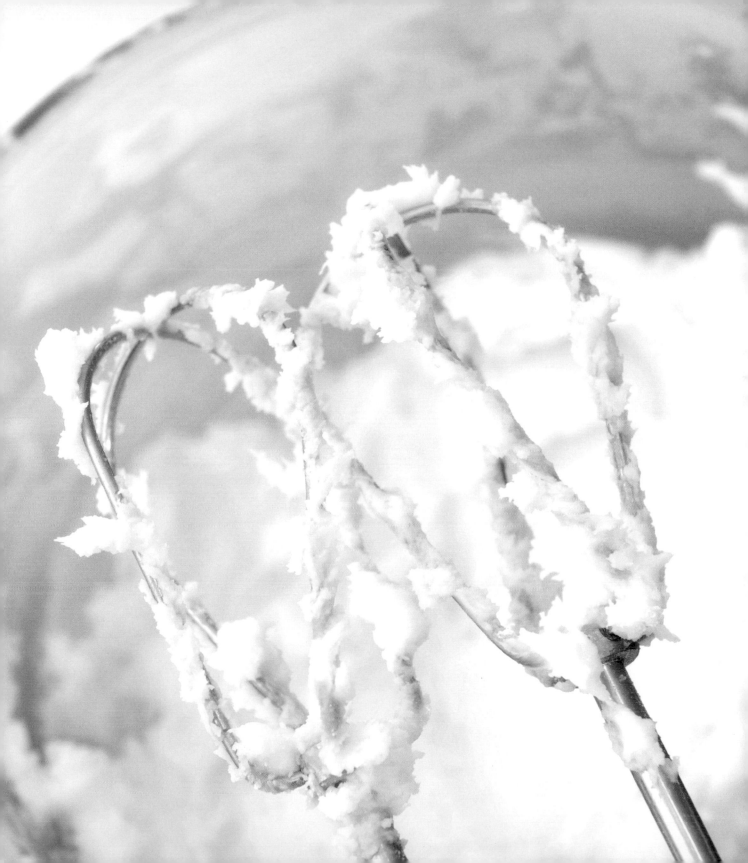

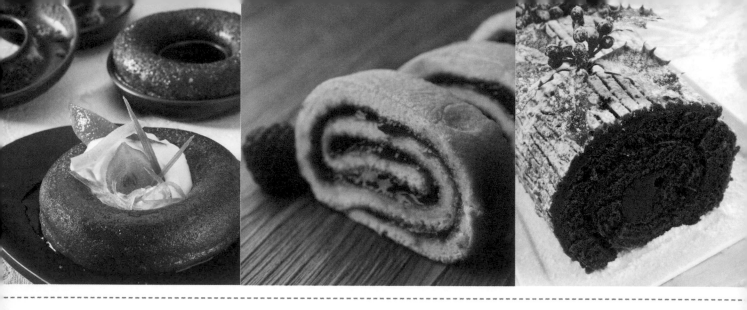

CHAPTER 2:

Cakes and Tortes to Tempt

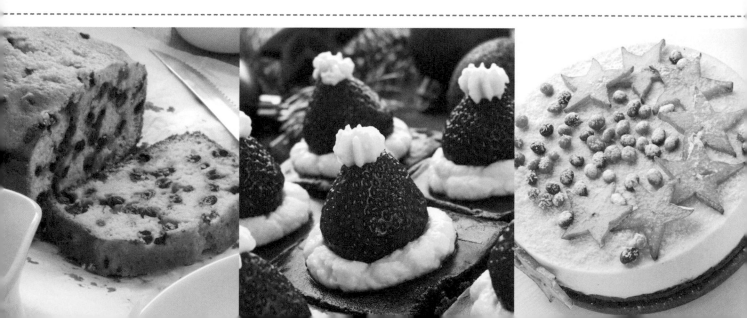

W hile we associate the cookie jar with the holidays, close at hand is the cake plate. Perhaps the most famous of all Christmas cakes is the French Yule log called a Bûche de Nöel, and you'll find a recipe for that showstopper in this chapter, along with a great variety of other luscious and rich desserts.

Baking Pan Sizes

It's always best to use the pan specified in a recipe. However, if that is not possible, the way to determine the best substitution is to know the capacity of pans. It really makes no difference if the pan is round or rectangular, as long as the correct amount of batter is added.

Use a liquid measuring cup and water to measure the volume of pans. Use this method as well for novelty pans such as hearts and Christmas trees.

Baking times and temperatures can change, however, with the dimensions of the pan. The best way to make adjustments is to look for a similar recipe specifying the size pan you are using.

Round Cake Pans	Volume	Pie Pans	Volume
8x1.5 inches	4 cups	8x1.25 inches	3 cups
9x1.5 inches	6 cups	9x1.5 inches	4 cups

Rectangular Cake Pans	Volume	Loaf Pans	Volume
8x 8x2 inches	6 cups	8.5x4.5x2.5 inches	6 cups
9x9x1.5 inches	8 cups	9x5x3 inches	8 cups
9x9x2 inches	10 cups		
13x9x2 inches	14 cups		

Apple and Gingerbread Upside-Down Cake

This variation on the theme of a cake with fruit on the bottom baked in a skillet is wonderful for fall and winter when apples are in season, and this cake stays moist for days. The gingerbread flavoring makes it festive, too.

Yield: 8 servings

Active time: 20 minutes

Start to finish: 1¼ hours

2 Red Delicious apples

¾ cup (1½ sticks) unsalted butter, softened, divided

1¼ cups firmly packed light brown sugar, divided

¾ cup brown rice flour

½ cup potato starch

¼ cup tapioca flour

1½ teaspoons baking soda

1 teaspoon ground cinnamon

1 teaspoon ground ginger

¾ teaspoon xanthan gum

¼ teaspoon ground cloves

¼ teaspoon salt

1 cup molasses

1 cup boiling water

1 large egg, lightly beaten

Vanilla ice cream (optional)

1. Preheat the oven to 350°F. Slice apples vertically into thin slices through the core. Melt ¼ cup (½ stick) butter in a 10-inch cast iron or other ovenproof skillet over medium heat. Reduce heat to low, and sprinkle ¾ cup brown sugar evenly over butter; then cook, without stirring, for 3 minutes. Not all of sugar will dissolve. Remove the skillet from the heat and arrange apple slices close together on top of brown sugar.

2. Whisk together brown rice flour, potato starch, tapioca flour, baking soda, cinnamon, ginger, xanthan gum, cloves, and salt in a mixing bowl. Whisk together molasses and boiling water in a small bowl. Combine remaining ½ cup (1 stick) butter, remaining ½ cup brown sugar, and egg in a large bowl. Beat with an electric mixer on medium speed for 2 minutes or until light and fluffy.

3. Reduce mixer speed to low, and add flour mixture in 3 batches, alternating with molasses mixture, beginning and ending with flour mixture. Beat until just combined. Gently spoon batter over apples, and spread evenly.

4. Bake cake for 40–45 minutes, or until golden brown and a cake tester inserted in the center comes out clean. Run a thin knife around the edge of the skillet. Wearing oven mitts, immediately invert a serving plate over the skillet and, holding the skillet and plate together firmly, invert them. Carefully lift off the skillet. If necessary, replace any fruit that might have stuck to the bottom of the skillet on top of the cake. Cool at least 15 minutes or to room temperature before serving, and serve with vanilla ice cream, if using.

Note: The cake can be baked up to 8 hours in advance and kept at room temperature.

Variation:
* *Substitute pears for the apples.*

> **Cinnamon is the inner bark of a tropical evergreen tree that's harvested during the rainy season and then allowed to dry. At that time it's sold as sticks or ground. What we call cinnamon is cassia cinnamon, and there's also a Ceylon cinnamon that is less pungent.**

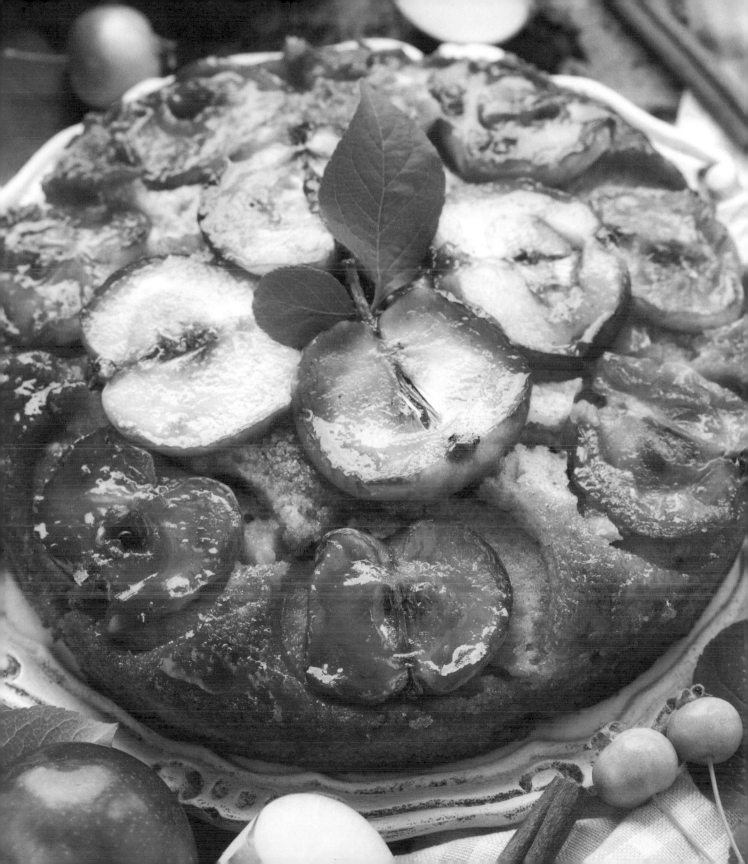

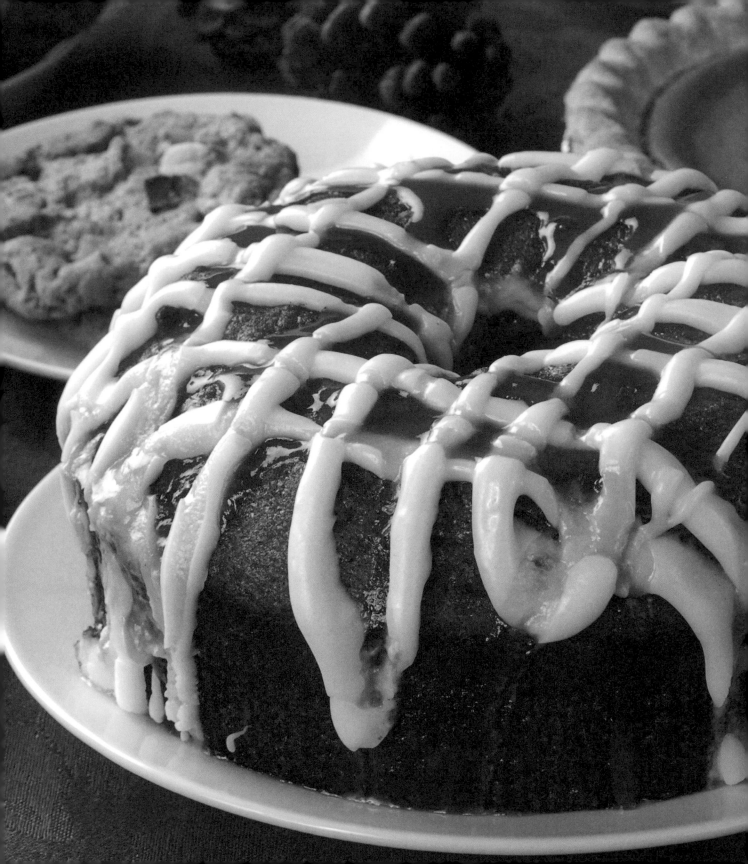

Spiced Apple Cake

This moist cake has the same wonderful apple flavor as a pie, but it's hand-holdable and feeds a lot of people too. The fruit flavor is enhanced by aromatic Chinese five-spice powder.

Yield: 10–12 servings

Active time: 20 minutes

Start to finish: 2 hours, including time for cooling

¾ cup raisins

⅓ cup rum, divided

½ cup (1 stick) unsalted butter, melted and cooled

2 large eggs, at room temperature

1 cup granulated sugar

2 teaspoons Chinese five-spice powder

1½ teaspoons gluten-free baking powder

¾ teaspoon xanthan gum

½ teaspoon salt

¾ cup brown rice flour

½ cup potato starch

¼ cup tapioca flour

3 Granny Smith apples

1 cup confectioners' sugar

3 tablespoons dark rum

1. Preheat the oven to 350°F. Grease a 10-inch bundt pan and dust it with brown rice flour. Combine raisins and ¼ cup rum in a small microwave-safe bowl, and heat on High (100 percent) power for 45 seconds. Stir, and allow raisins to plump.

2. Combine butter, eggs, sugar, five-spice powder, baking powder, xanthan gum, and salt in a mixing bowl. Whisk by hand until smooth. Add brown rice flour, potato starch, and tapioca flour, and stir well; the batter will be very thick.

3. Peel, quarter, and core apples. Cut each apple quarter in half lengthwise, and then thinly slice apples. Add apples to batter, and stir to coat apples evenly. Pack batter into the prepared pan.

4. Bake cake in the center of the oven for 1 hour, or until a toothpick inserted in the center comes out clean. Cool cake in the pan set on a rack for 20 minutes, or until cool. Invert cake onto a serving platter.

5. Combine confectioners' sugar and remaining rum in a small bowl. Drizzle glaze over top of cake, allowing it to run down the sides. Serve immediately.

Note: The cake can be prepared up to 1 day in advance and kept at room temperature, loosely covered with plastic wrap.

Variations:
* *Substitute apple pie spice or pumpkin pie spice for the Chinese five-spice powder.*
* *Substitute ripe pears for the apples.*

There isn't really an Aunt Jemima or a Jolly Green Giant, but there certainly was a Johnny Appleseed. Named John Chapman, he was born in Massachusetts in 1774. Unlike the artistic depictions of him propagating apples by tossing seeds out of his backpack, Chapman actually started nurseries for European species of apple brought from England as seedlings in the Allegheny Valley in 1800. By the time of his death in 1845, he had pushed as far west as Indiana, establishing groves of apple trees.

Gingered Apricot Torte

The gingered sugar on top of this moist and rich torte enlivens the flavor of the succulent fruit. Here is one treat that is at home both on a festive brunch table and after dinner.

Yield: 6–8 servings

Active time: 15 minutes

Start to finish: 1½ hours

4 ripe apricots

⅔ cup white rice flour

¼ cup potato starch

3 tablespoons tapioca flour

1 teaspoon baking powder

½ teaspoon xanthan gum

Pinch of salt

½ cup (1 stick) unsalted butter, softened

1¼ cups granulated sugar, divided

2 large eggs, at room temperature

¼ cup finely chopped crystallized ginger

½ teaspoon ground ginger

1. Preheat the oven to 350°F. Grease a 9-inch springform pan and dust it with rice flour.

2. Rinse apricots, and cut each into 6 slices. Whisk together rice flour, potato starch, tapioca flour, baking powder, xanthan gum, and salt.

3. Combine butter and 1 cup sugar in another mixing bowl and beat at low speed with an electric mixer to combine. Increase the speed to high, and beat for 3–4 minutes, or until light and fluffy. Beat in eggs, one at a time, beating well between each addition. Add flour mixture and crystallized ginger, and mix until just combined.

4. Scrape batter into the prepared pan, and smooth top. Arrange apricot slices on top of batter. Combine remaining sugar and ginger. Sprinkle over apricots.

5. Bake for 1 hour, or until a toothpick inserted in the center comes out clean. Remove torte from the oven and cool in the pan on a wire rack. Remove from the pan, and serve.

Note: The torte can be prepared up to 2 days in advance and kept at room temperature, tightly covered. It can also be frozen for up to 2 months.

Variations:
* *Substitute plums or pears for the apricots.*
* *Substitute firmly packed light brown sugar and cinnamon for the granulated sugar and ginger.*

> **Crystallized ginger is fresh ginger that is preserved by being candied in sugar syrup. It's then tossed with coarse sugar. It's very expensive in little bottles in the spice aisle, but most whole foods markets sell it in bulk.**

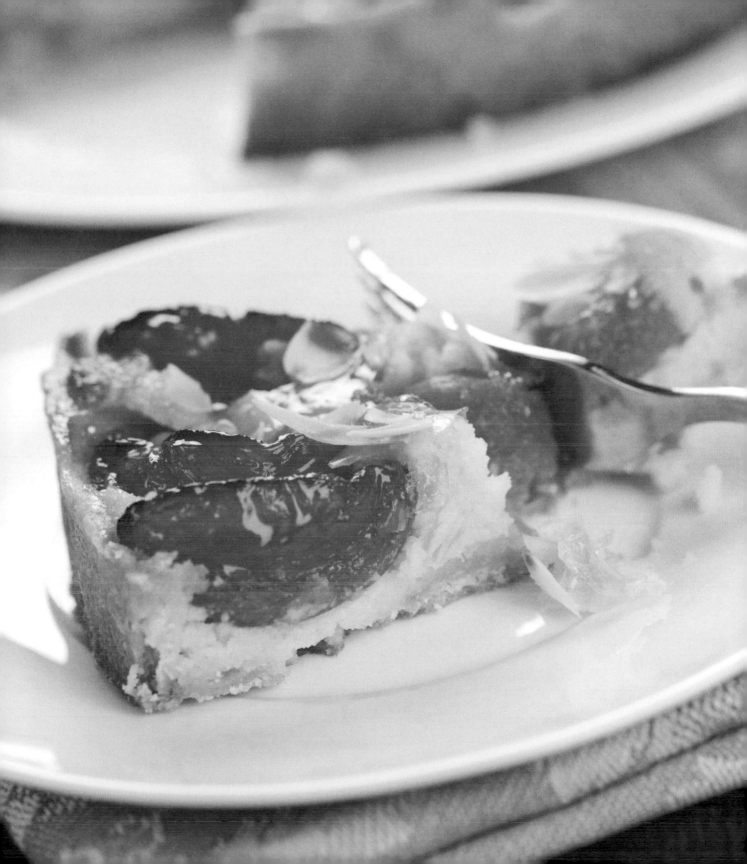

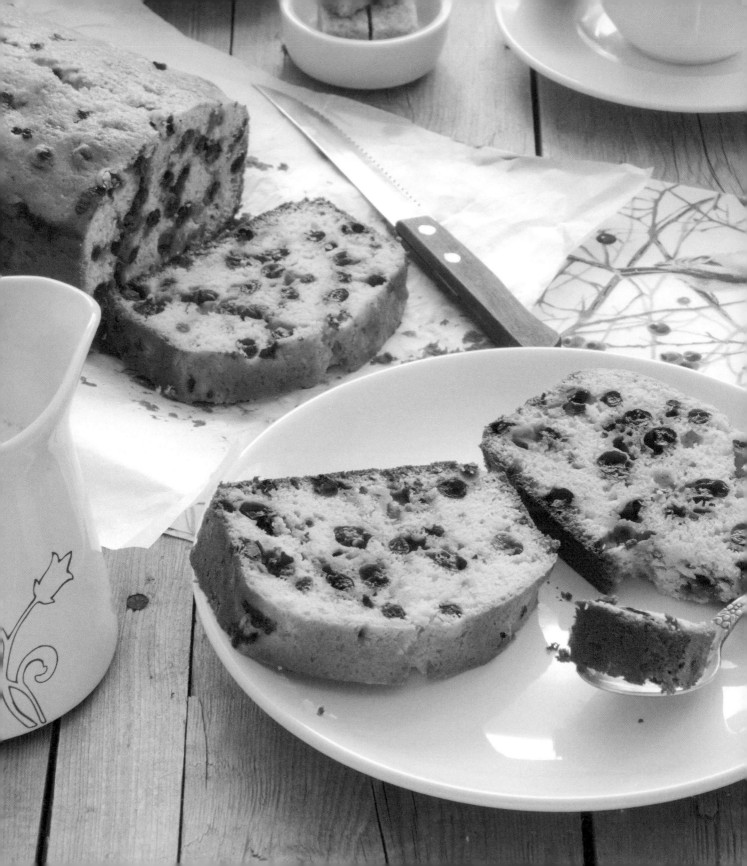

Cranberry Cake

Although we associate cranberry sauce with Thanksgiving, the cranberry is actually in season well into January, and its bright color and tart flavor make it a wonderful star for this cake too.

Yield: 10–12 servings

Active time: 15 minutes

Start to finish: 1½ hours

1¼ cups potato starch

1 cup white rice flour

¾ cup tapioca flour

1½ teaspoons baking soda

½ teaspoon salt

1 teaspoon xanthan gum

1½ cups granulated sugar

¾ cup (1½ sticks) unsalted butter, melted and cooled

2 large eggs

2 teaspoons grated orange zest, divided

1¼ cups buttermilk

1½ cups fresh cranberries

1 cup dried cranberries

1 tablespoon freshly squeezed orange juice

½ cup confectioners' sugar

1. Preheat the oven to 350°F. Butter a 10-inch bundt pan and dust it with white rice flour.

2. Sift potato starch, white rice flour, tapioca flour, baking soda, salt, and xanthan gum together. Whisk sugar, ⅔ of butter, eggs, and 1 teaspoon orange zest together in a large bowl. Whisk in one-third of dry mixture, then one-third of buttermilk. Repeat twice more, until all ingredients are incorporated. Stir in fresh cranberries and dried cranberries and scrape the batter into the prepared pan.

3. Bake for 50 minutes, or until a toothpick inserted in the center comes out clean. Allow cake to cool on a rack for 10 minutes, then invert it onto the rack to cool completely.

4. To prepare icing, combine remaining butter, remaining orange zest, orange juice, and confectioners' sugar in a small bowl and stir well. Drizzle icing over cooled cake.

Note: The cake can be prepared 1 day in advance and kept covered at room temperature.

Variation:

❋ *Substitute fresh and dried sour cherries for the two forms of cranberries.*

> **Early colonist William Byrd wrote in his 1711 diary that he "said my prayers and ate some cranberry tart for breakfast." The cranberry, along with the blueberry and Concord grape, is one of North America's three native fruits that are still commercially grown. Native Americans—who discovered the wild berry's versatility as a food, fabric dye, and healing agent—first used cranberries.**

Cannoli Cheesecake

Cannolis are wonderful Italian pastries served during the holidays. A filling of sweetened ricotta is stuffed into crispy tubes of fried dough. The same group of ingredients, including miniature chocolate chips and pistachio nuts, flavor this rich and delicious cheesecake.

Yield: 8–12 servings

Active time: 20 minutes

Start to finish: 6 hours, including time to chill

1 cup crumbs made from Gluten-Free Graham Crackers (page 60)

½ cup finely chopped pistachios

4 tablespoons (½ stick) unsalted butter, melted

⅔ cup granulated sugar, divided

1 (15-ounce) container whole-milk ricotta

1 tablespoon grated orange zest

1 large egg, at room temperature, separated

½ teaspoon pure orange oil

⅔ cup finely chopped candied fruit

⅓ cup miniature chocolate chips

2 tablespoons potato starch

4 large egg whites, at room temperature

Pinch of salt

¼ teaspoon cream of tartar

1 cup Royal Icing (page 17)

For garnish: Candied cherry halves, shaved bittersweet chocolate, and coarsely chopped pistachio nuts

1. Preheat the oven to 350°F. Grease the bottom and sides of a 9-inch springform pan.

2. Combine crumbs, nuts, butter, and 3 tablespoons sugar in a mixing bowl, and stir well. Pat mixture onto bottom and ½ inch up the sides of the prepared pan. Bake crust for 8–10 minutes, or until lightly browned.

3. Combine ricotta, remaining sugar, orange zest, egg yolk, and orange oil in a mixing bowl, and beat at medium speed with an electric mixer for 2 minutes. Combine chopped fruit, chocolate chips, and potato starch in a bowl, and toss to coat evenly. Fold into ricotta mixture.

4. Place all 5 egg whites in a grease-free mixing bowl and beat at medium speed with an electric mixer until frothy. Add salt and cream of tartar, raise the speed to high, and beat until soft peaks form. Add remaining sugar, 1 tablespoon at a time, and continue to beat until stiff peaks form and meringue is glossy. Fold meringue into ricotta mixture.

5. Bake in the center of the oven for 50–55 minutes, or until top is brown. Cool cake in the pan on a rack, and then refrigerate until cold. Run a knife around the sides of the pan to release cake, and then remove sides of pan.

6. Spread top of chilled cake with Royal Icing, allowing it to drip down the sides. Decorate top of cake with cherries, chocolate shavings, and pistachios. Allow cheesecake to sit at room temperature for 30 minutes before serving.

Note: The cake can be made up to 4 days in advance and refrigerated, tented with plastic wrap. Allow it to sit at room temperature for 30 minutes before serving.

Variation:
✷ *Substitute chopped toasted almonds for the pistachios, pure almond extract for the orange oil, omit the orange zest, and add 2 tablespoons amaretto liqueur to the ricotta mixture.*

> **To prevent cheesecakes from cracking on top, don't open up the oven door at all during the baking process. Most cracks are the result of drafts.**

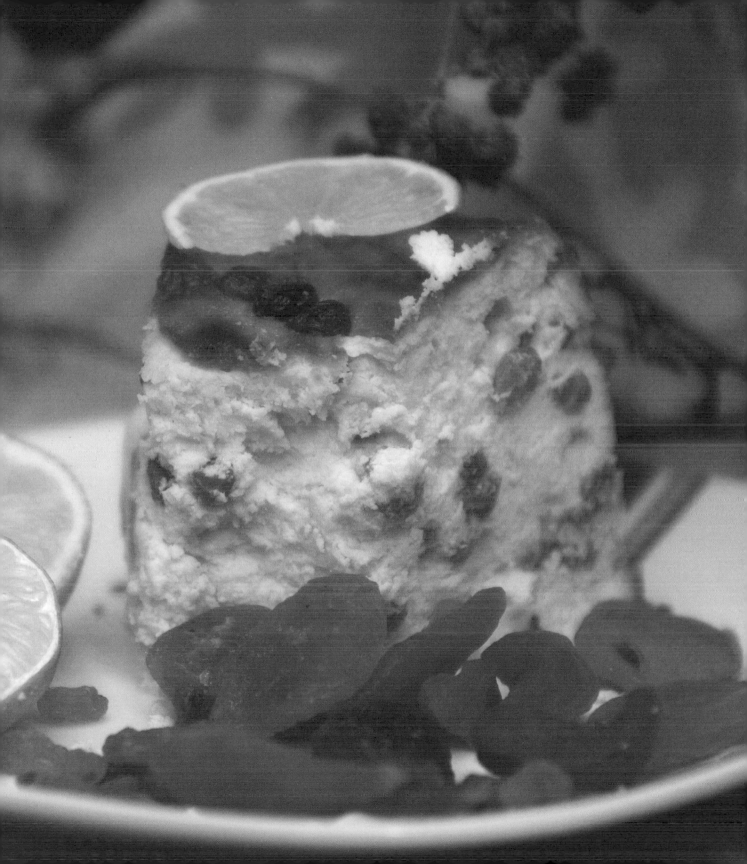

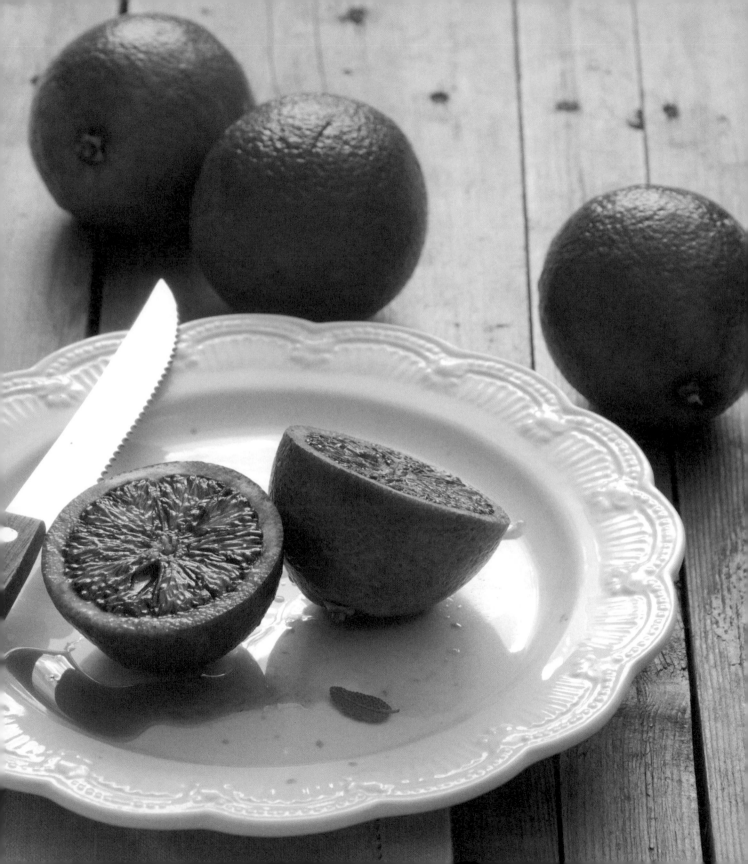

Hazelnut Orange Torte

Blood oranges, native to southern Italy, are now becoming commonplace here, and they add their tart-sweet flavor and blushing red color to this luscious torte.

Yield: 9–12 servings

Active time: 20 minutes

Start to finish: 1½ hours

2 blood oranges

7 ounces (1½ cups) skinned hazelnuts

½ cup potato starch

1 tablespoon gluten-free baking powder

½ teaspoon xanthan gum

Pinch of salt

¾ cup (1½ sticks) unsalted butter, melted

4 eggs, at room temperature, separated

⅔ cup granulated sugar, divided

½ teaspoon pure vanilla extract

½ teaspoon cream of tartar

Confectioners' Sugar Glaze (page 16)

1. Preheat the oven to 350°F. Grease a 9-inch square baking pan, line the pan with parchment paper, and grease the parchment paper. Grate zest off of oranges, and then squeeze juice. Set aside.

2. Grind hazelnuts in a food processor fitted with the steel blade until very fine. Transfer to a mixing bowl. Add potato starch, baking powder, xanthan gum, and salt to hazelnuts, and whisk well.

3. Combine orange juice, orange zest, butter, egg yolks, ¼ cup sugar, and vanilla extract in another bowl, and whisk well. Add to bowl with hazelnut mixture, and whisk until smooth.

4. Place egg whites in a grease-free bowl and beat at medium speed with an electric mixer until frothy. Add cream of tartar and continue beating, raising the speed to high, until soft peaks form. Continue beating, adding remaining sugar, 1 tablespoon at a time, until the meringue forms stiff peaks and is shiny. Gently fold meringue into the hazelnut mixture, being careful to avoid streaks of white meringue. Scrape batter into the prepared pan.

5. Bake in the center of the oven for 50 minutes, or until a toothpick inserted in the center comes out clean. Cool in the pan on a rack for 10 minutes. Invert cake onto the rack and discard parchment. Turn cake right side up and cool completely. Once cool, drizzle top with Confectioners' Sugar Glaze.

Note: Cake can be prepared up to 1 day in advance and kept at room temperature, tightly covered with plastic wrap.

Variations:
* *Substitute lemons or limes for the blood oranges.*
* *Substitute blanched almonds for the hazelnuts, and substitute pure almond extract for the vanilla extract.*

Skinning hazelnuts is not a fun task, so try to find them already skinned. If you have to do it yourself, bake them for 25 minutes, then place them in a towel and rub them back and forth. The skins will come off.

Lemon Polenta Cake

I always keep one of these cakes in the freezer, cut into slices, for emergency entertaining, because it freezes so well. The combination of the almond meal and polenta create a cake with a dense texture that's moist from the soaking syrup. Serve it with some sliced fruit.

Yield: 16 slices

Active time: 20

Start to finish: 1½ hours

2 lemons

2 cups almond meal

¾ cup gluten-free fine polenta

1½ teaspoons gluten-free baking powder

½ teaspoon xanthan gum

¼ teaspoon salt

14 tablespoons (1¾ sticks) unsalted butter, softened

1 cup granulated sugar

3 large eggs, at room temperature

1¼ cups confectioners' sugar

1. Preheat the oven to 350°F. Line the bottom of a 9-inch springform pan with parchment paper, and grease the parchment and sides of the pan. Grate zest and squeeze juice from lemons, and set aside separately.

2. Combine almond meal, polenta, baking powder, xanthan gum, and salt ion a mixing bowl, and whisk well.

3. Combine butter and sugar in another mixing bowl and beat at low speed with an electric mixer to combine. Increase the speed to High, and beat for 3–4 minutes, or until light and fluffy. Beat 1 egg into butter mixture, and then one-third of polenta mixture. Continue adding eggs and dry ingredients alternately, then beat in lemon zest.

4. Scrape batter into the prepared pan, and bake in the center of the oven for 40–45 minutes, or until a toothpick inserted into the center comes out with just a few crumbs attached and the cake starts to pull away from the sides of the pan. Transfer the cake to a cooling rack.

5. Combine lemon juice and confectioners' sugar in a small saucepan. Stir over low heat until sugar dissolves. Prick cake all over with a toothpick, and spoon warm syrup over cake. Cool completely, then remove cake from the pan.

Note: Cake can be prepared up to 1 day in advance and kept at room temperature, tightly covered with plastic wrap.

Variation:
* *Substitute blood oranges for the lemons.*

> **If your butter is too hard to blend, do not try to soften it in the microwave. A few seconds too long and you've got a melted mess. An easy way to soften butter quickly is to grate it through the large holes of a box grater. It will soften in a matter of minutes at room temperature.**

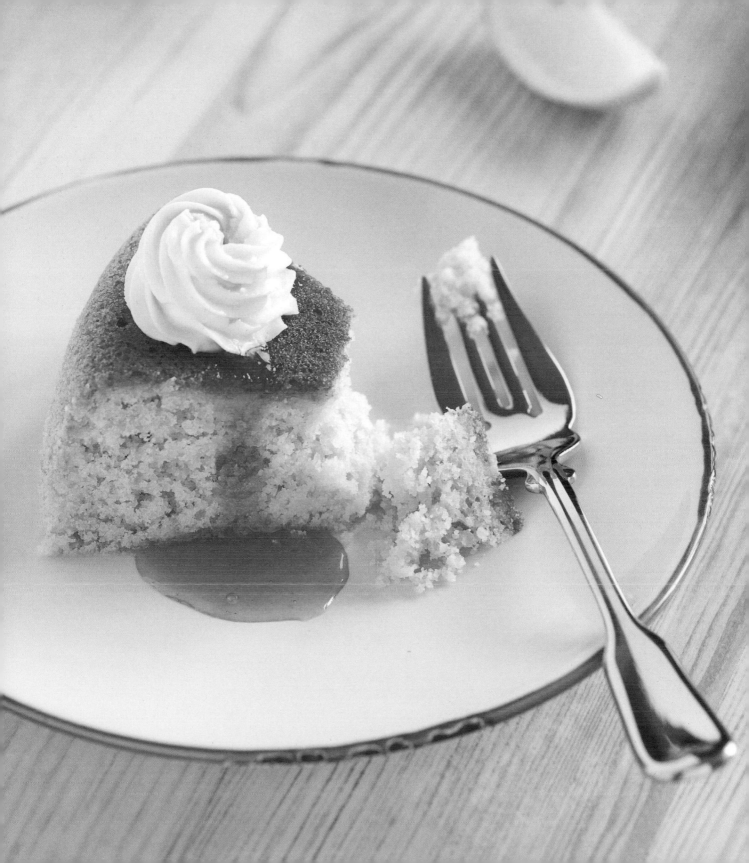

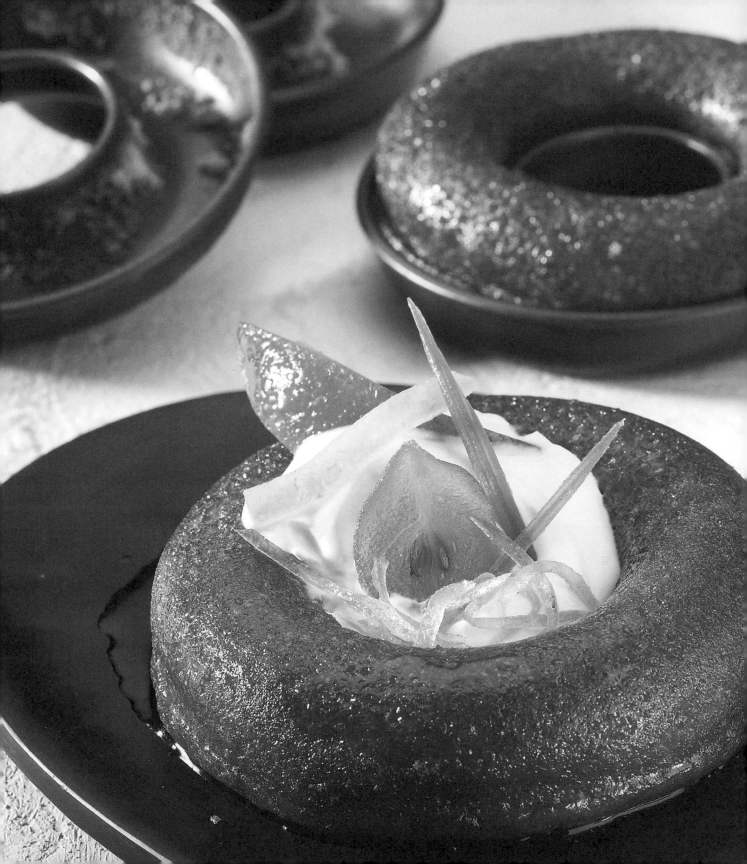

Baba au Rhum

This is clearly an adult cake; the rum is not cooked so it has its full alcohol content—although it's not enough to feel the effects. I usually serve it topped with some cooked blueberries or peaches.

Yield: 12–14 servings

Active time: 15 minutes

Start to finish: 2¼ hours

Cake

½ cup whole milk

4 teaspoons (2 envelopes) dry active yeast

⅔ cup brown rice flour

⅔ cup soy flour

½ cup tapioca flour

¼ cup whey powder

1 tablespoon granulated sugar

1½ teaspoons xanthan gum

3 large eggs, at room temperature

¼ pound (1 stick) unsalted butter, melted and cooled

Syrup

1 cup granulated sugar

1½ cups water

⅔ cup rum

½ teaspoon pure vanilla extract

1. Heat milk in a small saucepan to 110° F. Stir in yeast, and wait 2 minutes to allow yeast to soften. Combine brown rice flour, soy flour, tapioca flour, whey powder, sugar, and xanthan gum in a mixing bowl, and whisk well. In the bowl of a standard electric mixer, combine yeast mixture and ½ cup flour mixture. Stir to form a sponge and let rise, covered, until doubled, about 20 minutes.

2. Beating with the paddle attachment, add eggs 1 at a time, followed by remaining 1½ cups flour. When a soft dough forms, slowly beat in butter to make a smooth dough. Let rest for 15 minutes.

3. Grease and flour a large baba mold or 9-inch bundt cake pan. Place dough in the prepared pan, cover with plastic wrap, and let rise in a warm, draft-free place until it has nearly reached the top of the mold, about 40 minutes.

4. While baba rises, preheat the oven to 375°F. Bake baba on the middle rack of the oven for 30 minutes, or until the top is golden brown and the sides have begun to pull away from the pan slightly.

5. While baba bakes, make syrup. Place sugar and water in a small saucepan and cook over high heat until the sugar dissolves. Add rum and vanilla and set aside.

6. Remove baba from the oven, and cool on a wire rack for 10 minutes. Set the wire rack over a platter. Using a meat fork or long skewer, poke holes all over the top of the cake. Pour warm syrup over warm cake and let sit for 5 minutes, or until the liquid is absorbed. Turn baba out onto the wire rack, and let drain over the platter for 30 minutes; pour any accumulated syrup back onto cake.

Note: The cake can be made up to 3 days in advance and refrigerated, tightly covered. Allow it to reach room temperature before serving.

Variations:
* *Substitute triple sec or crème de cassis for the rum.*
* *Substitute 1 (6-ounce) can orange juice concentrate or lemon juice concentrate for the rum, and decrease the sugar to ½ cup.*

> **Baba au Ruhm has been found on menus in the New World since the late nineteenth century and is still the signature dessert of famed French chef Alain Ducasse.**

Coconut Rum Torte

I'm always in favor of a one-bowl recipe, and this fits the definition. No creaming of butter and sugar, no folding anything. Just whisk it together and you're done. And the result is a moist and rich cake with great coconut flavor, all topped with cream cheese frosting.

Yield: 8 servings

Active time: 20 minutes

Start to finish: 4 hours, including 2 hours for cake to cool

1½ cups sweetened coconut flakes

⅔ cup white rice flour

⅓ cup potato starch

¼ cup tapioca flour

1½ teaspoons baking powder

¾ teaspoon xanthan gum

¼ teaspoon salt

4 large eggs plus 3 large egg yolks

1½ cups granulated sugar

1½ teaspoons pure vanilla extract, divided

¾ cup (1½ sticks) unsalted butter, melted and cooled

½ cup well-stirred sweetened cream of coconut such as Coco López

½ cup dark rum

1 (8-ounce) package cream cheese, softened

3 cups confectioners' sugar

1 teaspoon grated lemon zest

1. Preheat the oven to 375°F with the rack in middle. Lightly grease a 9-inch round layer pan, and line the bottom with a round of parchment paper. Lightly grease the parchment paper, and then dust the inside of the pan with white rice flour, tapping out excess flour over the sink.

2. Bake coconut flakes on a baking sheet for 5–7 minutes, or until browned. Remove coconut from the oven, and set aside. Reduce the oven temperature to 350°F.

3. Whisk together white rice flour, potato starch, tapioca flour, baking powder, xanthan gum, and salt in a small bowl. Whisk together eggs, egg yolks, sugar, and 1 teaspoon vanilla in a large bowl, beating until mixture is thick and lemon-colored. Add ½ cup toasted coconut, flour mixture, and butter, and whisk until just combined. Pour batter into the prepared pan, and rap the pan on the counter to expel air bubbles.

4. Bake for 45 minutes, or until golden brown and cake starts to pull away from the side of the pan. Cool in the pan on a rack for 10 minutes. Invert cake onto the rack and discard parchment. Cool 10 minutes more.

5. Combine cream of coconut and rum in a small bowl, and stir well. Remove 3 tablespoons of mixture, and set aside. Using a meat fork, poke holes in the bottom of cake, and brush coconut rum mixture on the bottom. Allow it to soak in, and repeat. Turn cake over on the rack, and slice off the top so it is level. Spread remaining coconut rum mixture on top, and allow it to soak in. Allow cake to cool completely.

6. For icing, combine cream cheese, confectioners' sugar, remaining ½ teaspoon vanilla, lemon zest, and reserved coconut rum mixture in a food processor fitted with the steel blade. Process until smooth, and scrape into a bowl. Apply frosting to cake, and pat remaining 1 cup toasted coconut on the top.

Note: The cake can be baked and soaked with the coconut rum mixture up to 2 days in advance and kept at room temperature, tightly covered with plastic wrap. The cake can be frosted up to 1 day in advance and kept at room temperature, lightly covered.

Variation:
* *Substitute Grand Marnier, triple sec, or other orange-flavored liqueur for the rum.*

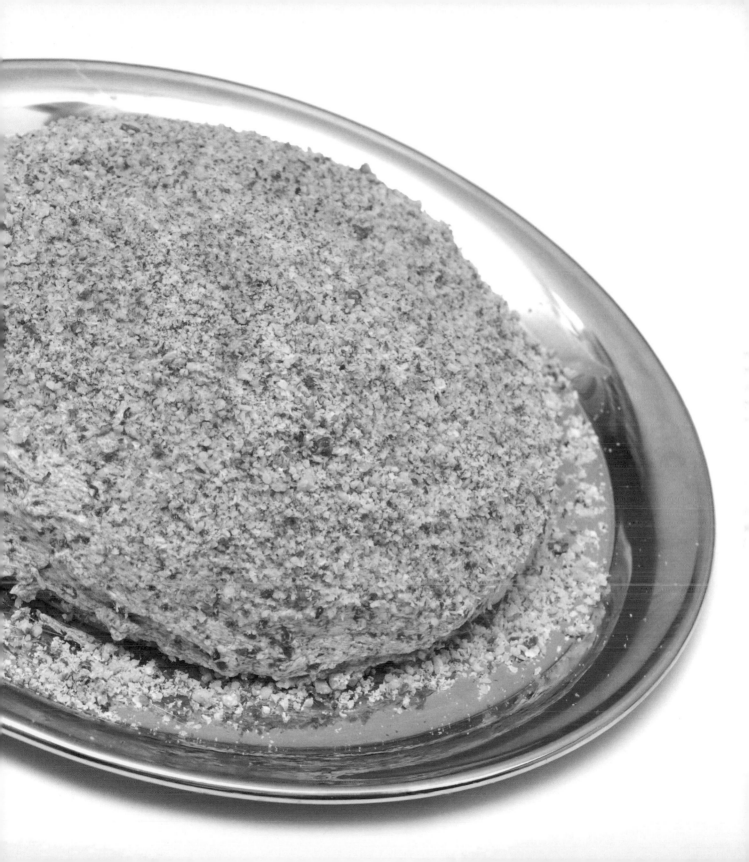

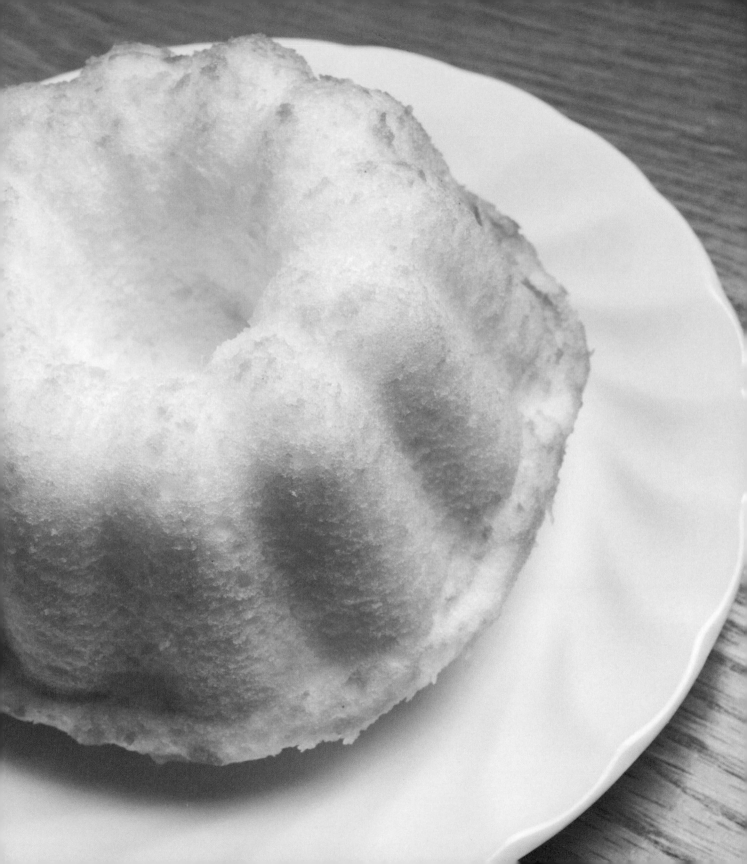

Citrus Angel Food Cake

The tangy tastes of orange and lemon are consistent with the light, airy quality of angel food cake. This cake can serve as the base for many mixed fruit salads, as well as being delicious all alone.

Yield: 8 servings

Active time: 25 minutes

Start to finish: 2½ hours

¾ cup orange juice

2 tablespoons finely grated orange zest

2 tablespoons finely grated lemon zest

⅓ cup potato starch

⅓ cup white rice flour

¼ cup tapioca flour

½ teaspoon xanthan gum

¾ cup granulated sugar, divided

10 large egg whites, at room temperature

1 teaspoon cream of tartar

1. Preheat the oven to 350°F. Rinse a tube pan and shake it over the sink to remove excess moisture, but do not wipe it dry.

2. Combine orange juice, orange zest, and lemon zest in a small heavy saucepan and bring to a boil over medium heat. Reduce by three-quarters, pour mixture into a soup bowl, and refrigerate until cool. Sift potato starch, white rice flour, tapioca flour, and xanthan gum with ¼ cup of sugar; set aside.

3. Place egg whites in a grease-free mixing bowl and beat at medium speed with an electric mixer until frothy. Add cream of tartar, raise the speed to high, and beat until soft peaks form. Add remaining sugar, 1 tablespoon at a time, and continue to beat until stiff peaks form and meringue is glossy. Lower the speed to Low and beat in cooled orange juice mixture. Gently fold flour mixture into meringue and scrape batter into the tube pan.

4. Bake in the center of the oven for 40–45 minutes, then remove cake from the oven and invert cake onto the neck of a tall bottle for at least 1½ hours, or until cool. Run a knife or spatula around the outside of the pan to loosen cake and invert cake onto a serving plate.

Note: Cake can be prepared up to 1 day in advance and kept at room temperature, tightly covered with plastic.

Variation:
✳ *Substitute lime zest for the lemon zest.*

> Egg white is very high in protein, with almost no fat, and virtually no cholesterol. It has merely 13 percent of the calories of a whole egg, and the other nutrient in egg whites is B-2 or riboflavin.

Almond Jellyroll Cake

Jellyrolls look dramatic on the table, and the actual cake is really light too. This gluten-free version is made with almond meal, which adds its tantalizing nutty flavor to the cake.

Yield: 8–10 servings

Active time: 20 minutes

Start to finish: 2 hours, including time for cake to cool

½ cup white rice flour

⅓ cup almond meal

⅓ cup potato starch

½ teaspoon xanthan gum

½ teaspoon gluten-free baking powder

¼ teaspoon salt

5 large eggs, at room temperature, and separated

¼ teaspoon cream of tartar

¾ cup superfine granulated sugar, divided

1 teaspoon pure almond extract

¼ cup confectioners' sugar

1 cup strawberry preserves, stirred well

1. Preheat the oven to 350°F. Line a 10x15-inch jellyroll pan with parchment paper, and grease the paper.

2. Sift white rice flour, almond meal, potato starch, xanthan gum, baking powder, and salt into a mixing bowl. Set aside.

3. Place egg whites in a grease-free mixing bowl and beat at medium speed with an electric mixer until frothy. Add cream of tartar, raise the speed to high, and beat until soft peaks form. Add ¼ cup sugar, 1 tablespoon at a time, and continue to beat until stiff peaks form and meringue is glossy.

4. Beat egg yolks at high speed with an electric mixer until thick and lemon colored. Gradually add remaining sugar, and beat for 3 minutes. Beat in flour mixture, almond extract, and one-fourth of meringue. Fold in remaining meringue, being careful to avoid streaks of white meringue. Spread batter evenly in the prepared pan.

5. Bake in the center of the oven for 15–18 minutes, or until cake springs back when touched lightly.

6. Spread a clean cloth kitchen towel on the counter, and sprinkle the towel with confectioners' sugar. Invert cake onto the towel. Discard parchment paper. Trim off crisp edges with a sharp serrated knife. Spread preserves evenly over cake. Roll cake and towel into a 5-inch roll. Cool completely on a cooling rack with the seam side down. Serve at room temperature or slightly chilled.

Note: The cake can be completed 1 day in advance and kept at room temperature, lightly covered with plastic wrap.

Variations:
* *Substitute pure orange oil for the almond extract, and add 2 tablespoons grated orange zest to the cake batter. Substitute orange marmalade for the strawberry preserves.*
* *Substitute raspberry or blueberry preserves for the strawberry preserves.*

> **Eggs should always be at room temperature when using them in baking, since the whites will not increase in volume properly if they are chilled. An easy way to do this is to place the eggs in a bowl of very hot tap water for 5 minutes before separating them.**

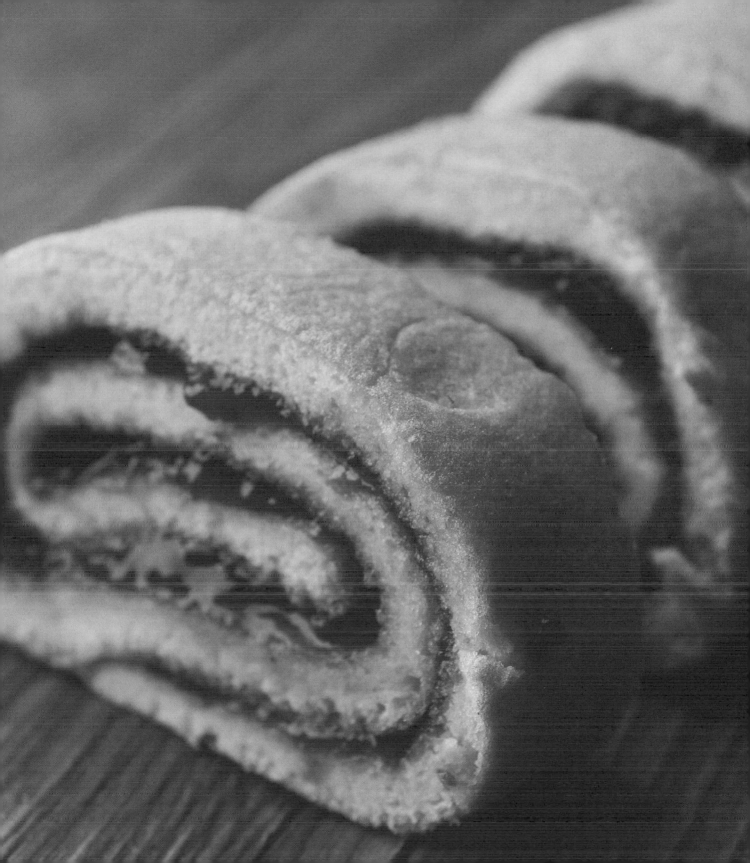

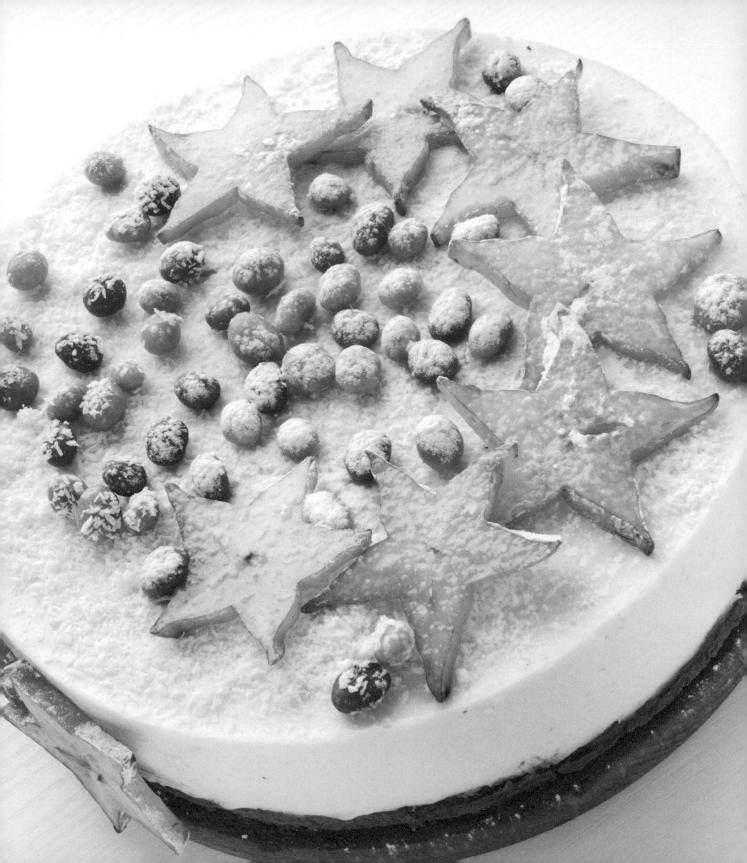

Cheesecake

Cheesecake is a perennial favorite—at the holidays or at any time of the year. You can top it with fruit or a fruit sauce, or just enjoy it.

Yield: 12–16 servings

Active time: 20 minutes

Start to finish: 6 hours, including time to chill

1½ cups crumbs made from Gluten-Free Graham Crackers (page 60)

5 tablespoons unsalted butter, melted

2 cups granulated sugar, divided

4 (8-ounce) packages cream cheese, softened

2 tablespoons white rice flour

2 tablespoons tapioca flour

4 large eggs, at room temperature

2 large egg yolks, at room temperature

1 teaspoon pure vanilla extract

Pinch of salt

1. Preheat the oven to 500°F.

2. Combine crumbs, butter, and ⅓ cup sugar in a mixing bowl, and stir well. Pat mixture into bottom and 1 inch up the sides of a 12-inch springform pan. Set aside.

3. Combine remaining sugar, cream cheese, rice flour, and tapioca flour in a large mixing bowl, and beat at medium speed of an electric mixer until smooth. Add eggs and egg yolks, 1 at a time, beating well between each addition, and scraping the sides of the bowl as necessary. Beat in vanilla and salt. Scrape mixture into the pan on top of crust.

4. Bake in the center of the oven for 15 minutes. Reduce the oven temperature to 225°F and continue to bake cheesecake for an additional 1 hour. Turn off the oven, and allow cheesecake to sit in the oven for an additional 30 minutes without opening the oven door.

5. Cool cake in the pan on a rack, and then refrigerate until cold. Run a knife around the sides of the pan to release cake, and then remove sides of pan. Allow cheesecake to sit at room temperature for 30 minutes before serving.

Note: Cheesecake lasts forever! You can refrigerate this cake for up to a week; keep it tightly covered with plastic wrap.

Variations:
* *Add 1 tablespoon grated lemon or orange zest to the batter.*
* *Substitute firmly packed dark brown sugar for the granulated sugar in the batter.*
* *Mix ¼ of the batter with 3 tablespoons unsweetened cocoa powder, and swirl this through the vanilla for a marble cheesecake.*

> When baking a cheesecake the center should still be a bit wobbly when you take it out of the oven. The residual heat will finish cooking it. This is the same reason that fish should be taken off the grill or broiler when it's slightly translucent in the center.

Chocolate Bûche de Nöel

This classic French cake shaped like a Yule log is truly the showstopper of any holiday meal. Rich chocolate buttercream is the filling and frosting for a chocolate jellyroll. You can become as creative as you'd like with the presentation by simply combing the frosting so that it resembles tree bark, to creating meringue mushrooms to surround it on the platter.

Yield: 10–12 servings

Active time: 40 minutes

Start to finish: 4 hours, including time to chill

Cake:

½ cup unsweetened cocoa powder

¼ cup cornstarch

3 tablespoons brown rice flour

½ teaspoon xanthan gum

½ teaspoon gluten-free baking powder

¼ teaspoon salt

5 large eggs, at room temperature, and separated

¼ teaspoon cream of tartar

⅔ cup superfine granulated sugar, divided

1 teaspoon pure vanilla extract

¼ cup confectioners' sugar

Filling and Frosting:

1 ¾ cups heavy whipping cream

1 cup (2 sticks) unsalted butter, sliced

3 tablespoons light corn syrup

1½ pounds bittersweet chocolate, chopped

1 teaspoon pure vanilla extract

Pinch of salt

1. Preheat the oven to 350°F. Line a 10x15-inch jellyroll pan with parchment paper, and grease the paper.

2. Sift cocoa powder, cornstarch, brown rice flour, xanthan gum, baking powder, and salt into a mixing bowl. Set aside.

3. Place egg whites in a grease-free mixing bowl and beat at medium speed with an electric mixer until frothy. Add cream of tartar, raise the speed to high, and beat until soft peaks form. Add ¼ cup sugar, 1 tablespoon at a time, and continue to beat until stiff peaks form and meringue is glossy.

4. Beat egg yolks at high speed with an electric mixer until thick and lemon colored. Gradually add remaining sugar, and beat for 3 minutes. Beat in cocoa mixture, vanilla, and one-fourth of meringue. Fold in remaining meringue, being careful to avoid streaks of white meringue. Spread batter evenly in the prepared pan.

5. Bake in the center of the oven for 15–18 minutes, or until cake springs back when touched lightly.

6. Spread a clean cloth kitchen towel on the counter, and sprinkle the towel with confectioners' sugar. Invert cake onto the towel. Discard parchment paper. Trim off crisp edges with a sharp serrated knife. Roll cake and towel into a 5-inch roll. Cool completely on a cooling rack with the seam side down.

7. Combine cream, butter, and corn syrup in a medium saucepan. Bring to a boil over medium heat, stirring frequently. Remove the pan from the heat, and add chocolate, vanilla, and salt. Whisk until smooth. Allow to stand at room temperature for 1½–2 hours, or until thick enough to spread.

8. Unroll cake, and spread with half of frosting. Reroll, and chill for 30 minutes, or until firm. Spread remaining frosting on the outside of the roll, and use a fork or decorating comb to create lines on frosting resembling tree bark.

Note: The cake can be completed 1 day in advance, tented with plastic wrap. Allow it to sit at room temperature for 30 minutes before serving.

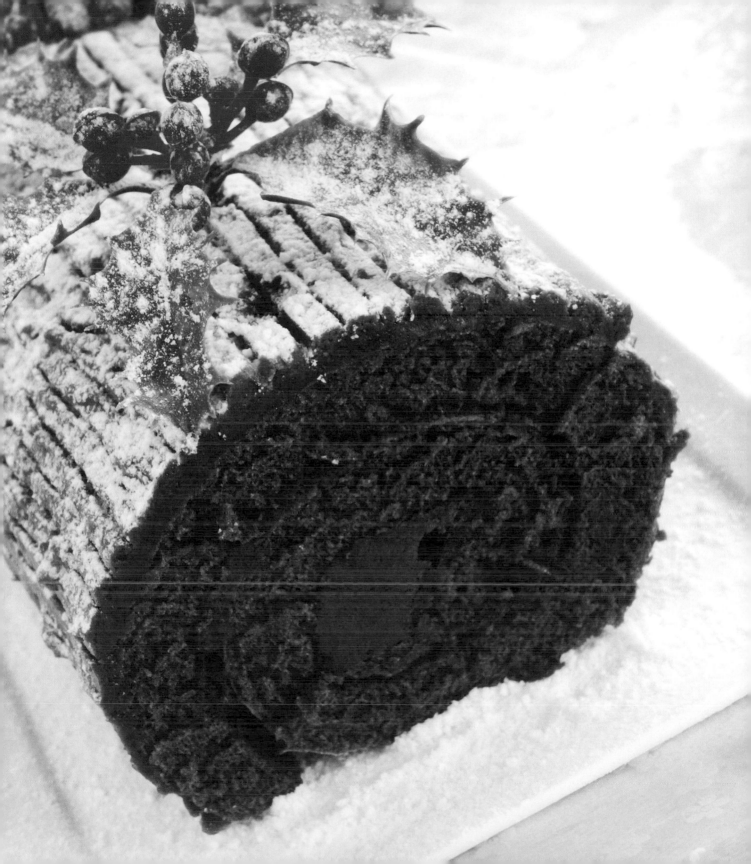

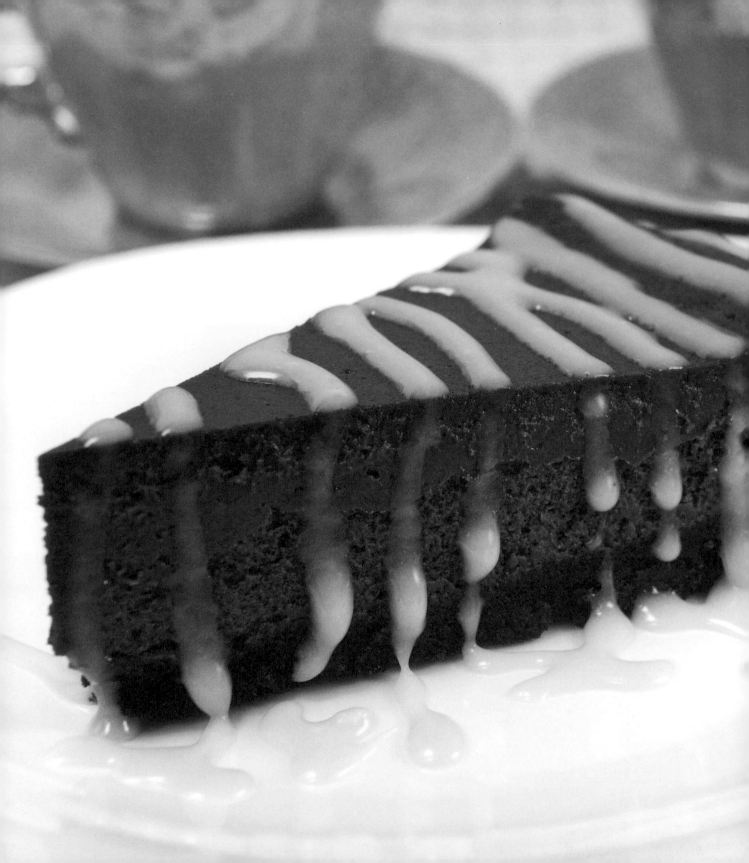

Chocolate Almond Cheesecake

Chocolate, cream cheese, and almonds are an unbeatable combination, especially in this dense and rich cheesecake.

Yield: 8–12 servings

Active time: 25 minutes

Start to finish: 6 hours, including time to chill

1 cup slivered blanched almonds

1½ cups crumbs from gluten-free chocolate cookies or Gluten-Free Graham Crackers (page 60)

¾ cup (1½ sticks) unsalted butter, melted, divided

9 ounces good-quality bittersweet chocolate, finely chopped, divided

2 (8-ounce) packages cream cheese, softened

½ cup sour cream

3 tablespoons amaretto or other almond-flavored liqueur

2 tablespoons brown rice flour

1 tablespoon potato starch

½ teaspoon pure almond extract

¼ teaspoon salt

2 large eggs, at room temperature

⅔ cup granulated sugar

1. Preheat the oven to 350°F. Grease the bottom and sides of a 9-inch springform pan. Place almonds on a baking sheet, and toast for 5–7 minutes, or until lightly browned. Remove the pan from the oven, and finely chop nuts in a food processor fitted with a steel blade, using on-and-off pulsing, or by hand.

2. Combine crumbs, 4 tablespoons butter, and 1 ounce chocolate in a mixing bowl, and stir well. Pat mixture onto bottom and ½ inch up the sides of the prepared pan. Bake crust for 8–10 minutes, or until lightly browned. Reduce the oven temperature to 325°F.

3. Melt remaining chocolate in remaining butter over low heat or in a microwave-safe bowl. Add cream cheese, sour cream, amaretto, rice flour, potato starch, almond extract, and salt. Beat for 1 minute on medium speed with an electric mixer.

4. Combine eggs and sugar in a mixing bowl. Beat for 3–4 minutes at high speed with an electric mixer until very thick and lemon colored. Fold in chocolate mixture and almonds.

5. Scrape mixture into the prepared pan. Bake for 1½ hours, or until top is brown. Cool cake in the pan on a rack, and then refrigerate until cold. Run a knife around the sides of the pan to release cake, and then remove sides of pan.

Note: The cake can be made up to 4 days in advance and refrigerated, covered with plastic wrap. Allow it to sit at room temperature for 30 minutes before serving.

Variations:
* *Substitute Frangelico or other hazelnut liqueur and roasted hazelnuts for the amaretto and almonds and substitute pure vanilla extract for the almond extract.*
* *Substitute Grand Marnier, triple sec, or other orange liqueur for the amaretto, pure orange oil for the almond extract, and ⅔ cup candied orange rind for the almonds.*

Because chocolate can absorb aromas and flavors from other foods, it should always be wrapped tightly after being opened. Store chocolate in a cool, dry place, but it should not be refrigerated or frozen. If stored at a high temperature, the fat will rise to the surface and become a whitish powder called a bloom. It will disappear, however, as soon as the chocolate is melted.

Flourless Chocolate Nut Torte

The batter for this luscious chocolate cake is created in a matter of minutes in a food processor. It's a dense and rich cake that is crunchy with nuts and topped with a candy-like ganache.

Yield: 8 servings

Active time: 15 minutes

Start to finish: 1½ hours, including 1 hour for chilling

10 ounces bittersweet chocolate, chopped, divided

2 cups pecan or walnut halves, toasted in a 350°F oven for 5 minutes

1 cup (2 sticks) unsalted butter, softened, divided

2 tablespoons plus ½ cup granulated sugar

3 large eggs, at room temperature

1 tablespoon rum

1. Preheat the oven to 375°F. Grease an 8-inch round cake pan, cut out a circle of waxed paper or parchment to fit the bottom, and grease the paper.

2. Melt 4 ounces chocolate in a microwave oven or over simmering water in a double boiler. Cool slightly. Reserve 12 nut halves and chop the remaining nuts with 2 tablespoons sugar in a food processor fitted with a steel blade, using on-and-off pulsing. Scrape nuts into a bowl. Beat ½ cup (1 stick) of butter and remaining ½ cup sugar in the food processor until light and fluffy. Add melted chocolate, then add eggs, 1 at a time. Beat well between each addition, and scrape the sides of the work bowl with a rubber spatula. Add rum, then fold chocolate mixture into ground nuts.

3. Scrape batter into the prepared pan and bake for 25 minutes. Cake will be soft but will firm up as it cools. Remove cake from the oven and cool 20 minutes on a rack. Invert cake onto a plate, remove the paper, and cool completely.

4. To make glaze, combine remaining 6 ounces chocolate and remaining ½ cup (1 stick) butter in a small saucepan. Melt over low heat and beat until shiny and smooth. Place cake on a rack over a sheet of wax paper. Pour the glaze onto the center of the cake, and rotate the rack at an angle so glaze runs down sides of the cake. Top with the nut halves, and allow to sit in a cool place until chocolate hardens.

Note: The cake can be prepared 1 day in advance and refrigerated. Allow it to reach room temperature before serving.

Variations:
* *Add 1 tablespoon instant espresso powder to the batter.*
* *Substitute Triple Sec or Grand Marnier for the rum, and add 2 teaspoons grated orange zest to the batter.*
* *Substitute blanched almonds for the pecans or walnuts, substitute amaretto for the rum, and add ½ teaspoon pure almond extract to the batter.*

If you find that the parchment paper sticks to the bottom of the cake, brush the paper with a little warm water. After ten seconds the paper will peel right off.

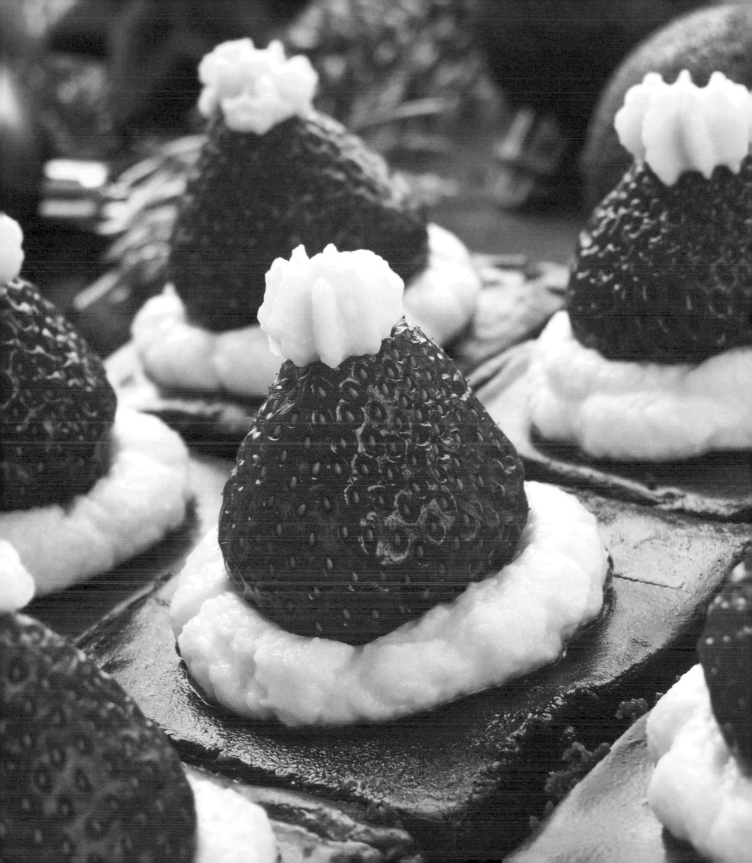

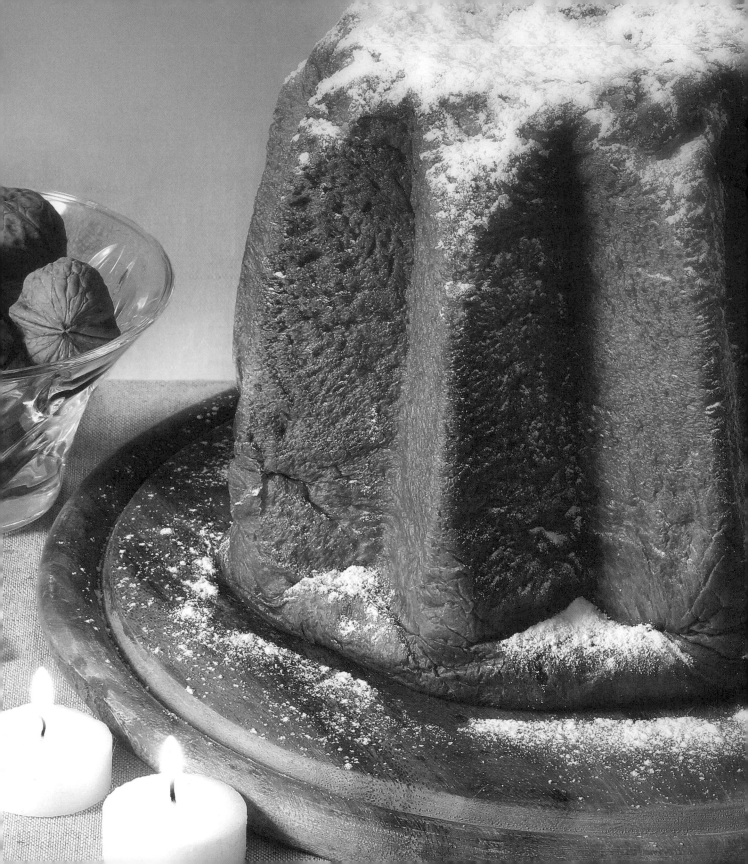

Chocolate Angel Food Cake

Light and airy angel food cake takes very well to being flavored with cocoa powder, and cocoa powder delivers a lot of chocolate flavor for very few calories. Top this cake with fruit salad or a more indulgent treat such as chocolate mousse.

Yield: 8 servings

Active time: 20 minutes

Start to finish: 2½ hours

5 tablespoons unsweetened cocoa powder (not Dutch processed)

⅓ cup potato starch

⅓ cup white rice flour

¼ cup tapioca flour

½ teaspoon xanthan gum

¾ cup granulated sugar, divided

10 large egg whites, at room temperature

¾ teaspoon cream of tartar

1 teaspoon pure vanilla extract

1. Preheat the oven to 350°F. Rinse out a tube pan and shake it over the sink, but do not wipe it dry. Set aside.

2. Sift together cocoa, potato starch, white rice flour, tapioca flour, and xanthan gum with ¼ cup of sugar. Set aside.

3. Place egg whites in a grease-free bowl and beat at medium speed with an electric mixer until frothy. Add cream of tartar and continue beating, raising the speed to high, until soft peaks form. Continue beating, adding remaining sugar, 1 tablespoon at a time, until meringue forms stiff peaks and is shiny. With the mixer at the lowest speed, beat in vanilla. Gently fold cocoa mixture into egg whites, being careful to avoid streaks of white meringue. Scrape batter into the tube pan.

4. Bake in the center of the oven for 40–45 minutes. Remove cake from the oven and invert the pan onto the neck of a tall bottle for at least 1½ hours, or until cool. Run a knife or spatula around the outside of the pan to loosen cake and invert cake onto a serving plate.

Note: Cake can be prepared up to 1 day in advance and kept at room temperature, tightly covered with plastic wrap.

Variations:
* *Dissolve 1 tablespoon instant espresso powder in 2 tablespoons boiling water, and beat it into batter along with the vanilla for a mocha cake.*
* *Substitute pure almond extract for the vanilla, and add ¾ teaspoon ground cinnamon to the batter.*

> **Cocoa powder has a tendency to become lumpy if exposed to humidity, and if you find that this is the case with your cocoa powder, sift the cocoa or shake it through a fine-meshed sieve before using it.**

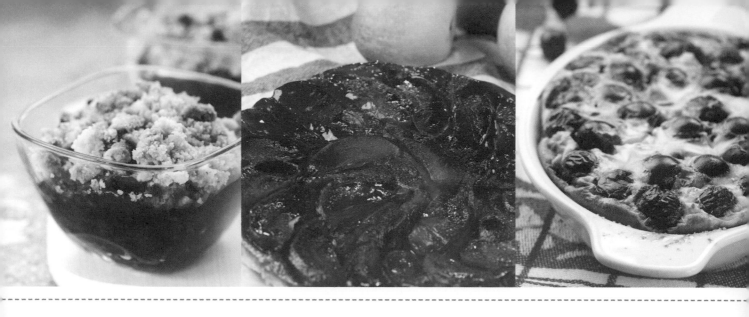

CHAPTER 3:

Pies and Pastries to Perk the Palate

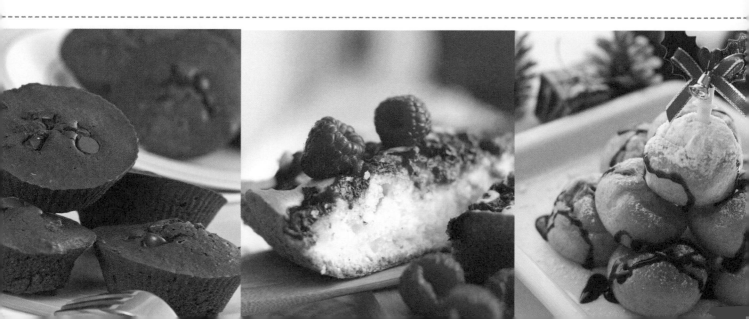

Most traditional fruit pies are thickened with cornstarch or tapioca, both of which are acceptable in a gluten-free diet. The problem with pies is the wheat flour in the crust rather than the filling. But the recipes in this chapter will change all of that.

The chapter begins with a few recipes for basic crusts that can be used for pies, tarts, and turnovers. If you omit the small amount of sugar, you can also use them for quiches and other savory pies. After those essential recipes, which are really the building blocks for thousands of desserts, there are some specific pies and pastries I like a lot for the holidays.

This chapter ends with a few miscellaneous desserts, including a homey cobbler, elegant chocolate tarts, and profiteroles.

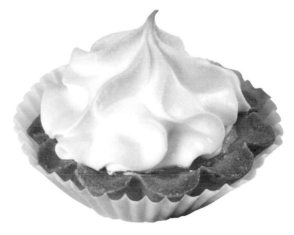

Basic Gluten-Free Piecrust

A benefit of gluten-free piecrust is that without gluten the result is always tender and flaky. The use of egg in the dough strengthens the dough in the same way as gluten so that the pies hold together.

Yield: Enough for 1 (8 or 9-inch) double crust pie

Active time: 15 minutes

Start to finish: 15 minutes

2 cups brown rice flour

1½ cups potato starch

½ cup tapioca flour

¼ cup granulated sugar

1 teaspoon xanthan gum

½ teaspoon salt

¾ cup (1½ sticks) unsalted butter, chilled

2 large eggs

⅓ cup ice water

1. Combine brown rice flour, potato starch, tapioca flour, sugar, xanthan gum, and salt in a mixing bowl, and whisk well. Cut butter into cubes the size of lima beans, and cut into dry ingredients using a pastry blender, two knives, or your fingertips until mixture forms pea-sized chunks. This can also be done in a food processor fitted with the steel blade using on-and-off pulsing.

2. Combine egg with ice water in a small bowl, and whisk well. Sprinkle mixture over dough, 1 tablespoon at a time. Toss lightly with fork until dough will form a ball. If using a food processor, process until mixture holds together when pressed between two fingers.

3. Depending on if it is to be a 1- or 2-crust pie, form dough into 1 or 2 (5 to 6-inch) "pancakes." Dust "pancakes" lightly on both sides with brown rice flour, and refrigerate dough for at least 30 minutes, and for up to 2 days.

4. Either roll dough between 2 sheets of waxed paper or inside a jumbo plastic bag that has been lightly dusted with brown rice flour. Use the former method for piecrust dough that will be used for formed pastries such as empanadas and the latter to make circles suitable for lining or topping a pie pan. For a round circle, make sure dough starts out in the center of the bag, and then keep turning it in ¼ turns until the circle is 1-inch larger in diameter than the inverted pie plate. Either remove the top sheet of wax paper or cut the bag open on the sides. You can either begin to cut out shapes or invert the dough into a pie plate, pressing it into the bottom and up the sides and extending the dough 1 inch beyond the edge of the pie plate.

5. If you want to partially or totally bake the pie shell before adding a filling, prick bottom and sides with a fork, press in a sheet of waxed paper or aluminum foil, and fill the pie plate with dried beans, rice, or metal pie stones sold in cookware stores. Bake crust in a 375°F oven for 10–15 minutes. The shell is now partially baked. To complete baking, remove the weights and liner, and bake for an additional 15–20 minutes, or until golden brown. Otherwise, fill pie shell. If you want a double crust pie, roll out the second dough "pancake" the same way you did the first half, and invert it over the top, crimping the edges and cutting in some steam vents with the tip of a sharp knife.

Note: The crust can be prepared up to 3 days in advance and refrigerated, tightly covered. Also, both dough "pancakes" and rolled out sheets can be frozen for up to 3 months.

Variation:
* *Omit the sugar for a neutral crust appropriate for quiche or other savory tartes.*

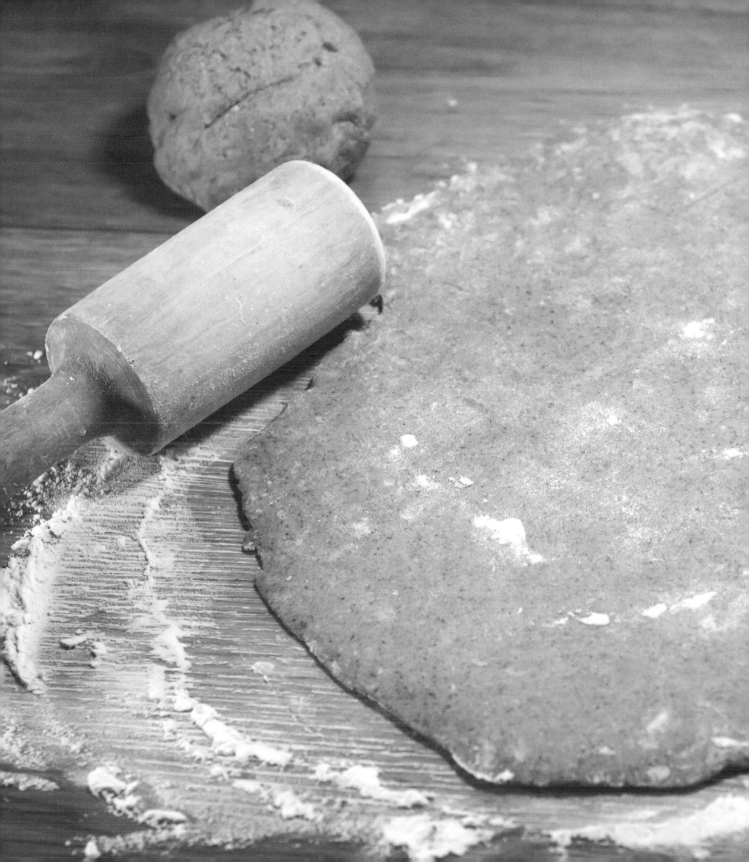

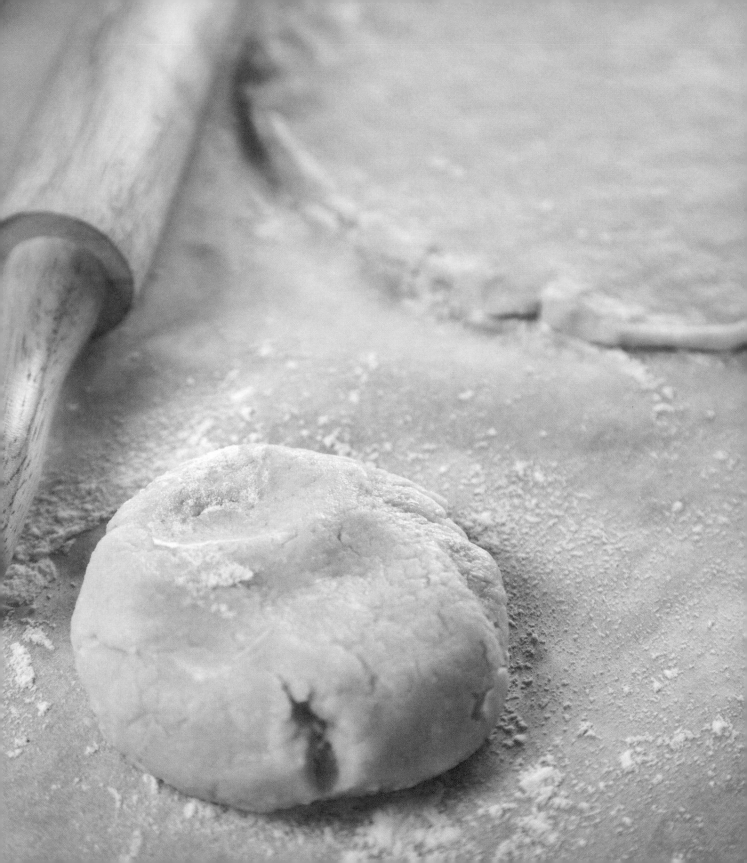

Almond Piecrust

This is my favorite crust recipe for fruit pies. It's sweetened with marzipan, and the aroma and flavor of the almonds melds beautifully with all sorts of fruit.

Yield: Enough for 1 (8 or 9-inch) double crust pie

Active time: 15 minutes

Start to finish: 15 minutes

1½ cups brown rice flour

1½ cups potato starch

½ cup tapioca flour

½ cup almond meal

½ teaspoon xanthan gum

½ teaspoon salt

1 (7-ounce) can marzipan

¾ cup (1½ sticks) unsalted butter, chill

1 large egg

2 tablespoons ice water

½ teaspoon pure almond extract

1. Combine brown rice flour, potato starch, tapioca flour, almond meal, xanthan gum, and salt in a mixing bowl, and whisk well. Place mixture in a food processor fitted with the steel blade, and break marzipan into small cubes. Process until crumbly.

2. Cut butter into cubes the size of lima beans, and cut into dry ingredients using a pastry blender, two knives, or your fingertips until mixture forms pea-sized chunks. This can also be done in a food processor fitted with the steel blade using on-and-off pulsing.

3. Combine egg, ice water, and almond extract in a small bowl, and whisk well. Sprinkle mixture over dough, 1 tablespoon at a time. Toss lightly with fork until dough will form a ball. If using a food processor, process until mixture holds together when pressed between two fingers.

4. Depending on if it is to be a 1- or 2-crust pie, form dough into 1 or 2 (5 to 6-inch) "pancakes." Dust "pancakes" lightly on both sides with brown rice flour, and refrigerate dough for at least 30 minutes, and for up to 2 days.

5. Either roll dough between 2 sheets of waxed paper or inside a jumbo plastic bag that has been lightly dusted with brown rice flour. Use the former method for piecrust dough that will be used for formed pastries such as empanadas, and the latter to make circles suitable for lining or topping a pie pan. For a round circle, make sure dough starts out in the center of the bag, and then keep turning it in ¼ turns until the circle is 1 inch larger in diameter than the inverted pie plate. Either remove the top sheet of wax paper or cut the bag open on the sides. You can either begin to cut out shapes or invert the dough into a pie plate, pressing it into the bottom and up the sides, and extending the dough 1 inch beyond the edge of the pie plate.

6. If you want to partially or totally bake the pie shell before adding a filling, prick bottom and sides with a fork, press in a sheet of waxed paper or aluminum foil, and fill the pie plate with dried beans, rice, or metal pie stones sold in cookware stores. Bake crust in a 375°F oven for 10–15 minutes. The shell is now partially baked. To complete baking, remove the weights and liner, and bake for an additional 15–20 minutes, or until golden brown. Otherwise, fill pie shell. If you want a double crust pie, roll out the second dough "pancake" the same way you did the first half, and invert it over the top, crimping the edges and cutting in some steam vents with the tip of a sharp knife.

Note: The crust can be prepared up to 3 days in advance and refrigerated, tightly covered. Also, both dough "pancakes" and rolled out sheets can be frozen for up to 3 months.

Gluten-Free Graham Crackers

You need graham crackers to form the basis for graham cracker crusts, which are so good with confections like key lime pies and cheesecakes. The proportions of crumbs to butter and additional sugar changes from recipe to recipe in this book, so what I'm giving you here are the basic crackers. You can use them to make S'mores, too.

Yield: 16–20, depending on size

Active time: 20 minutes

Start to finish: 1¾ hours

1½ cups brown rice flour

½ cup cornstarch

⅓ cup firmly packed dark brown sugar

1 teaspoon baking powder

¾ teaspoon xanthan gum

½ teaspoon ground cinnamon

½ teaspoon salt

6 tablespoons (¾ stick) unsalted butter, sliced

5 tablespoons whole milk

¼ cup honey

½ teaspoon pure vanilla extract

1. Combine rice flour, cornstarch, sugar, baking powder, xanthan gum, cinnamon, and salt in a food processor fitted with the steel blade. Blend for 5 seconds. Add butter to the work bowl, and process, using on-and-off pulsing, until mixture resembles coarse meal.

2. Combine milk, honey, and vanilla in a small cup, and whisk well. Drizzle liquid into the work bowl, and pulse about 10 times, or until stiff dough forms. If dough is dry and doesn't come together, add additional milk by 1-teaspoon amounts, until dough forms a ball.

3. Divide dough in half, and wrap each half in plastic wrap. Press dough into a pancake. Refrigerate dough for 1 hour or until firm, or up to 2 days.

4. Preheat the oven to 350°F. Line two baking sheets with parchment paper or silicone baking mats.

5. Lightly dust a sheet of waxed paper and a rolling pin with sweet rice flour. Roll each half of dough into a rectangle ¼-inch thick. Transfer dough to the prepared baking sheets, and cut each half into 8–10 rectangles with a pizza wheel. Prick dough all over with the tines of a fork.

6. Bake cookies for 15–17 minutes, or until browned. Allow cookies to cool completely on the cookie sheets placed on a wire cooling rack. Break cookies apart at scored lines.

Note: Keep cookies in an airtight container, layered between sheets of waxed paper or parchment, at room temperature for up to 5 days. Cookies can also be frozen for up to 2 months.

Variations:
* *Substitute ground ginger for the ground cinnamon.*
* *Sprinkle cookies with a mixture of ⅓ cup granulated sugar mixed with 1 teaspoon ground cinnamon before baking.*

> **When measuring sticky ingredients like honey or molasses, spray the measuring cup with vegetable oil spray. The sticky ingredient will slide right out of the cup.**

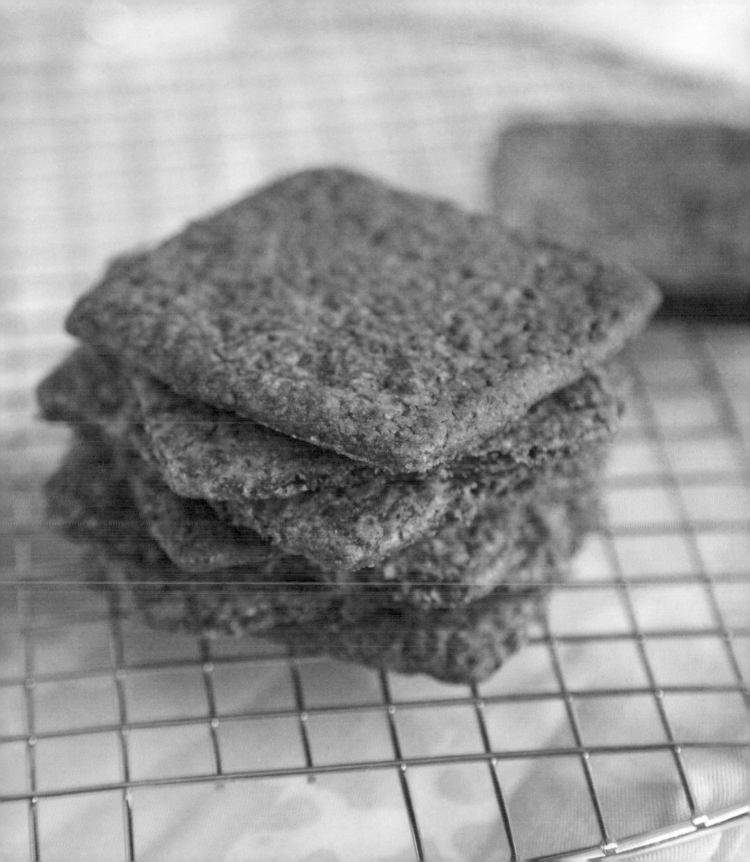

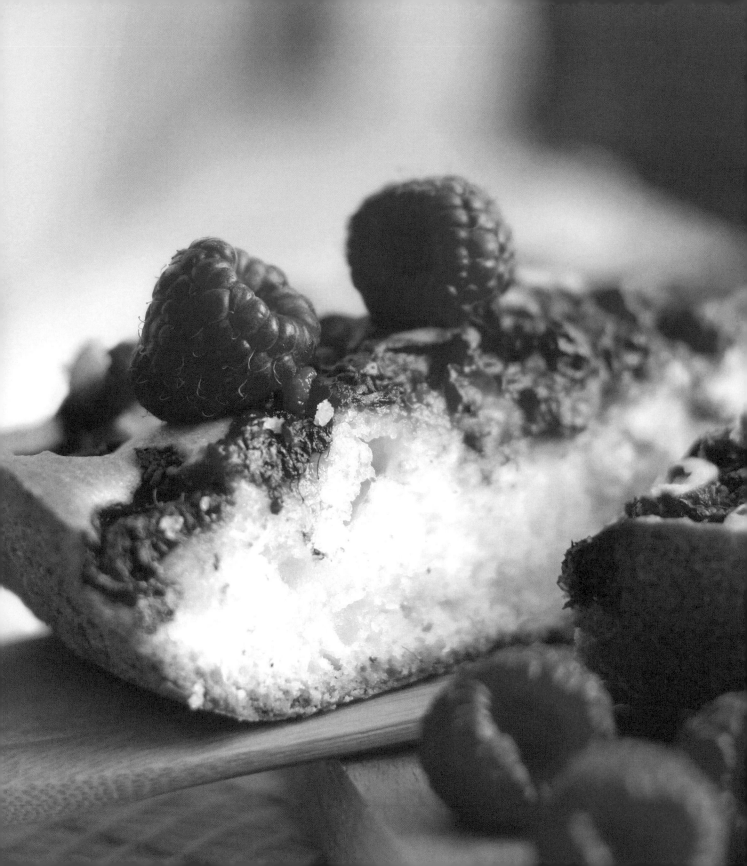

Raspberry Crème Fraîche Tart

Modern air transportation has given us a new definition of "airline food." We can now have bright red and sweet raspberries when there are snow drifts outside. The red berries give this sophisticated dessert a holiday feel, and it's very easy to make during a season when time is short.

Yield: 6 to 8 servings

Active time: 15 minutes

Start to finish: 3 hours, including time to chill

3 large eggs

½ cup granulated sugar

1 teaspoon pure vanilla extract

1¼ cups crème fraîche

1 pint fresh raspberries, rinsed

1 (9-inch) pre-baked pie shell made from Basic Gluten-Free Piecrust (page 56)

1. Preheat the oven to 350°F.

2. Whisk eggs and sugar in the top of a double boiler for 2 minutes, or until thick and lemon colored. Add vanilla and crème fraîche and stir well. Place mixture over water that is simmering in the bottom of the double boiler. Heat, stirring constantly, until the mixture is hot and starting to thicken.

3. Place raspberries in bottom of pie shell and pour warm custard over them. Bake for 10 minutes, or until the custard is set. Chill well before serving.

Note: The pie can be baked up to 1 day in advance and refrigerated, tightly covered.

Variations:
* *Substitute fresh blueberries or blackberries for the raspberries.*
* *Add 2 teaspoons grated orange zest to the custard, and substitute pure orange oil for the vanilla.*

When you're selecting boxes of fresh raspberries in the market, turn over the box and look at the paper on the bottom. It should not be stained red, which means the berries have been damaged and could be getting moldy.

Chocolate Caramel Pecan Pie

I believe that the first responsibility of any dessert is to contain at least some chocolate, and this pie is almost like eating a candy bar. It combines chocolate with crunchy pecans and mellow caramel.

Yield: 6 to 8 servings

Active time: 20 minutes

Start to finish: 1¾ hours, including time to cool

1½ cups granulated sugar

1 cup heavy cream

4 tablespoons (½ stick) unsalted butter, cut into small pieces

¼ cup bourbon

2 large eggs

1 cup pecan halves, toasted at 350°F for 5 minutes

4 ounces bittersweet chocolate, melted

1 (9-inch) pre-baked pie shell made from Basic Gluten-Free Piecrust (page 56)

1. Combine sugar and ⅓ cup water in a small saucepan and place over medium-high heat. Cook, without stirring, until liquid is golden brown and caramelized. Turn off the heat and add cream slowly, stirring with a long-handled spoon; it will bubble up at first. Once cream has been added, cook the caramel over low heat for 2 minutes. Strain the mixture into a mixing bowl and allow it to cool for 10 minutes.

2. Preheat the oven to 400°F.

3. Beat butter, bourbon, and eggs into caramel and whisk until smooth. Stir in pecans. Spread melted chocolate in bottom of pie shell and pour pecan filling over it. Bake for 15 minutes, then reduce the oven heat to 350°F and bake for an additional 15 minutes. Allow pie to cool on a wire rack until room temperature.

Note: The pie can be made 1 day in advance and refrigerated, tightly covered. Bring it to room temperature before serving.

Variations:
* *Substitute rum or brandy for the bourbon.*
* *Substitute walnuts, almonds, or pine nuts for the pecans.*

> **Caramelizing sugar is not difficult, but one pitfall is allowing the sugar to actually reach dark brown before removing the pan from the heat. The liquid and pot are very hot by the time the sugar starts to color, so take the pan off the heat when the syrup is a medium brown; it will continue to cook.**

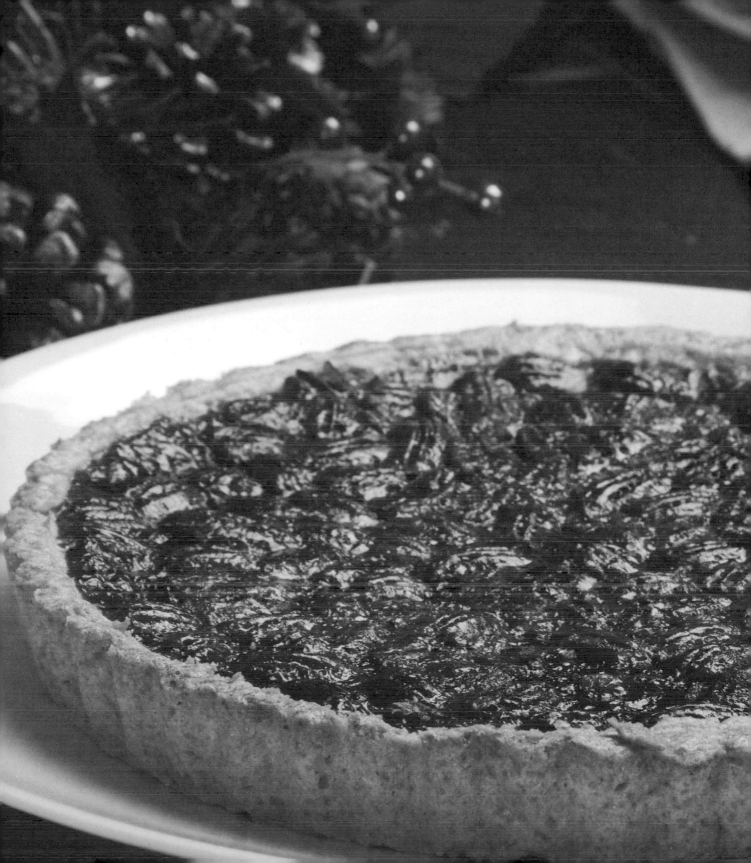

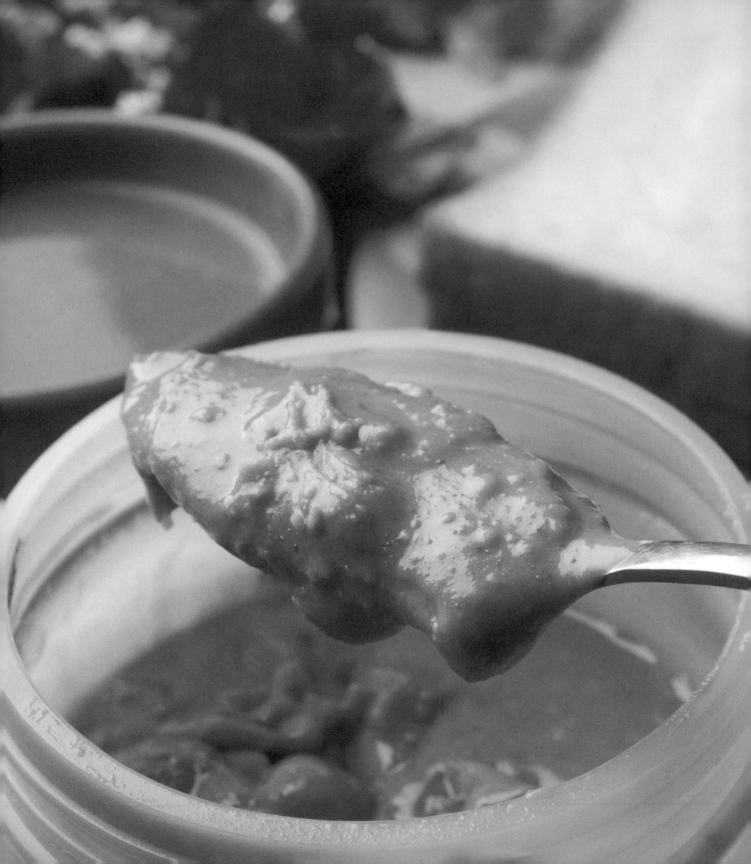

Peanut Butter Mousse Pie

The holidays are when many generations come together to celebrate, and this pie with its rich chocolate ganache layer topped by light mousse made with peanut butter is a favorite for children of all ages.

Yield: 8 to 10 servings

Active time: 20 minutes

Start to finish: 2 hours, including time to chill

1½ cups crumbs made from Gluten-Free Graham Crackers (page 60)

6 tablespoons unsalted butter, melted, divided

1 cup granulated sugar, divided

1 cup creamy commercial peanut butter

1 (8-ounce) package cream cheese, softened

1 teaspoon pure vanilla extract

1¾ cups heavy cream, divided

8 ounces bittersweet chocolate, chopped

1. Preheat the oven to 350°F. Combine crumbs, 5 tablespoons butter, and ¼ cup sugar in a mixing bowl, and mix well. Press mixture into the bottom and up the sides of a 9-inch pie plate. Bake crust for 8 to 10 minutes, or until lightly browned.

2. Beat peanut butter and remaining sugar with an electric mixer on medium speed until light and fluffy. Add cream cheese, remaining butter, and vanilla and beat well. In another mixing bowl, whip ¾ cup cream until medium-soft peaks form and fold it into peanut butter mixture until thoroughly combined. Refrigerate 30 minutes, or until slightly firm.

3. While mousse chills heat remaining cream to a boil over low heat. Add chocolate, and stir until melted and thoroughly combined. Pour chocolate into pie shell, reserving about ⅓ cup at room temperature. Chill until firmly set.

4. Remove mousse from the refrigerator. Beat with an electric mixer on low speed for at least 5 minutes, or until light and fluffy. Cover chocolate layer with peanut butter mousse and distribute it evenly with a spatula. Place remaining chocolate in a pastry bag fitted with the small tip or in a plastic bag with small hole at one corner. Drizzle it decoratively over mousse. Chill until ready to serve.

Note: The pie can be prepared 1 day in advance, and refrigerated.

Variation:
* *Substitute commercial almond butter for the peanut butter.*

> **To meet the standards set by the Food and Drug Administration, pure vanilla extract must contain about 1 pound vanilla beans per gallon; that's why it's about twice as expensive as imitation extract. It's clearly worth the money, considering how little you use. Look at the labels carefully before you buy.**

Upside-Down Caramel Apple Tart

This upside down pie, called a tarte tatin *in classic French cooking, is the ultimately showy apple dessert, but it's really quite easy to make. It's also speedier than a pie because the apples are basically cooked on top of the stove before a final baking.*

Yield: 6 to 8 servings

Active time: 20 minutes

Start to finish:
50 minutes

6 tablespoons (¾ stick)
unsalted butter

1½ cups granulated
sugar

6 Golden Delicious
apples, peeled, cored,
quartered, with
each quarter halved
lengthwise

3 tablespoons
lemon juice

½ teaspoon apple pie
spice

1 recipe Basic Gluten-
Free Pie Crust
(page 56)

1. Melt butter in 12-inch cast iron or other ovenproof skillet over medium-high heat. Stir in 1 cup sugar and cook, stirring frequently, for 6 to 8 minutes, or until syrup is a deep walnut brown. Remove pan from heat, and set aside.

2. Place apple slices in mixing bowl, and toss with remaining sugar, lemon juice, and apple pie spice. Allow to sit for 15 minutes.

3. Preheat the oven to 425°F. Drain apple slices, and arrange them tightly-packed in a decorative pattern on top of caramel. Place remaining apple slices on top of decorative base. Place pan over medium-high heat, and press down on the apples as they begin to soften.

4. Using a bulb baster, draw up juices from apples and pour juices over apples on the top. Do not stir apples. After 5 minutes, or when apples begin to soften, cover the pan, and cook apples for 10 to 15 minutes, or until apples are soft and liquid is thick. During this time continue to baste apples.

5. Take the pan off the heat, and form dough into a circle 1-inch larger than the circumference of the pan. Tuck ends around apples on the sides of the pan using the tip of a paring knife. Cut six (1-inch) slits in top of dough to allow for release of steam.

6. Bake tart for 20 minutes, or until pastry is golden and juices are thick. Remove the pan from the oven, and allow to cool for 10 minutes. Using a knife, loosen edges of tart from the pan. Invert a serving plate over the pan and then, holding the pan and the plate together firmly, invert them. Lift off the pan. Replace any apples that might have stuck to the bottom of the pan on top of the tart. Serve warm or at room temperature.

Note: The tart can be baked up to 6 hours in advance, and kept at room temperature.

Variation:
* *Substitute 6 ripe pears, peeled, cored, and sliced, for the apples.*

> **Apple pie spice is a combination of fragrant spices that are pre-blended, so you don't have to purchase all of them individually. You can make your own by combining ½ teaspoon cinnamon, ¼ teaspoon nutmeg, ⅛ teaspoon allspice, ⅛ teaspoon ground cardamom, and ¼ teaspoon ground cloves. Or, in a pinch, substitute cinnamon as the primary base, with a dash of any of the other spices you might have on hand.**

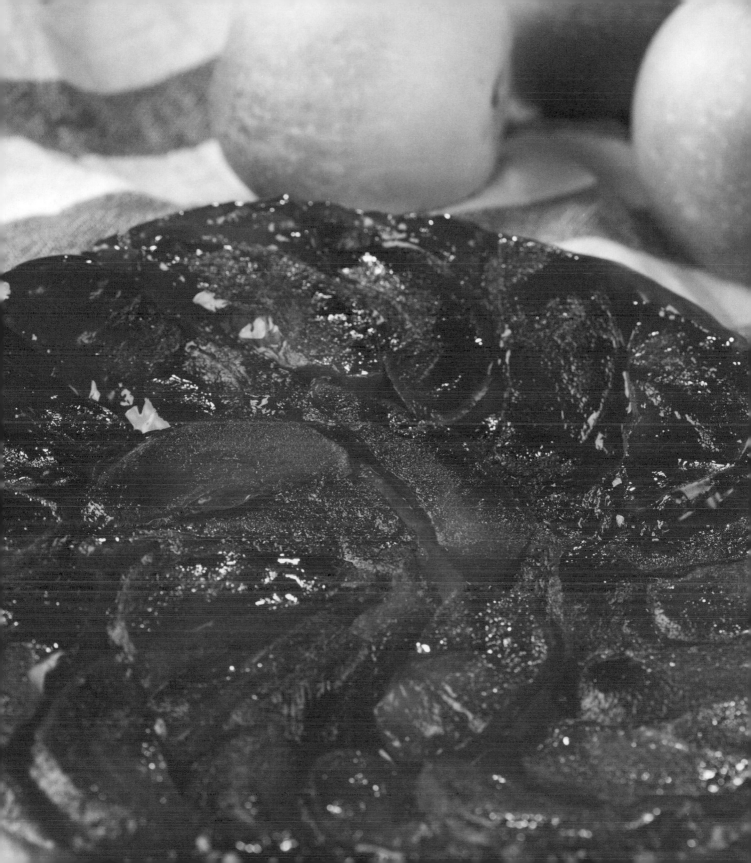

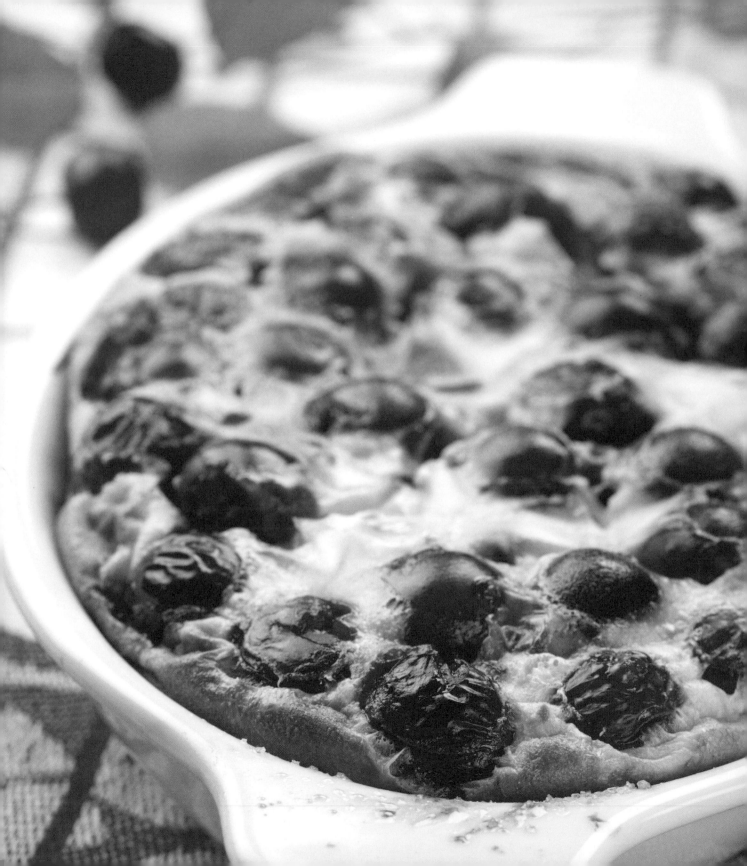

Plum Clafouti

Clafouti originated in the Limousin region of France. It is a very light dessert that combines fruit and a batter to produce a "cake" with the texture of a popover.

Yield: 6 to 8 servings

Active time: 10 minutes

Start to finish: 35 minutes

1 cup granulated sugar

¼ cup brown rice flour

2 tablespoons cornstarch

6 large eggs, at room temperature

2 cups whole milk

2 teaspoons pure vanilla extract

½ teaspoon salt

3 cups diced sweet ripe plums

2 tablespoons unsalted butter, cut into bits

Vanilla ice cream (optional)

1. Preheat the oven to 400°F, and grease a 9x13-inch baking pan.

2. Reserve 3 tablespoons sugar; combine remaining sugar, brown rice flour, cornstarch, eggs, milk, vanilla, and salt in a food processor fitted with a steel blade or in a blender. Puree until smooth.

3. Arrange plum pieces in 1 layer in the prepared baking pan, and pour custard over them. Bake for 20 to 25 minutes, or until top is puffed and springy to the touch. Remove the pan from the oven and increase the oven temperature to broil.

4. Sprinkle with remaining 3 tablespoons sugar, dot with butter, and broil clafouti under the broiler about 3-inches from the heat for 1 minute or until it is browned. Serve immediately with ice cream, if using.

Note: The batter can be prepared up to 1 day in advance and refrigerated, tightly covered. Do not bake the cake until just prior to serving.

Variation:
✳ *Any fruit that holds its shape and cooks in a relatively short amount of time is a candidate for this dessert. These include blueberries, sliced peaches, sliced apricots, and pitted sweet cherries.*

Brown & Polson in Paisley, Scotland, have been selling cornstarch, which they call cornflour, since 1840, and a man named Orlando Jones patented it in the US a year later. During the "Emergency," as the Irish called World War II, a special act was passed setting the maximum price for Brown & Polson Cornflour in Ireland at 5 pence a ¼ pound package.

Orange-Scented Cranberry and Apple Cobbler

I developed this recipe thinking about the cranberry-orange relish that my mother used to serve at Thanksgiving. It's a festive cobbler for all the fall and winter holidays, especially following turkey.

Yield: 8 servings

Active time: 20 minutes

Start to finish: 55 minutes

1 juice orange

3 cups fresh cranberries, picked over and rinsed

½ cup dried cranberries

1 cup granulated sugar, divided

1 cup cranberry juice cocktail

¼ cup Triple Sec or other orange-flavored liqueur

3 Golden Delicious or Granny Smith apples, peeled, cored, and cut into ½-inch slices

1 cup white rice flour

⅔ cup potato starch

⅔ cup tapioca flour

1 tablespoon gluten-free baking powder

½ teaspoon xanthan gum

½ teaspoon salt

2 large eggs, lightly beaten

¾ cup heavy cream

¼ cup sour cream

1. Preheat the oven to 375°F, and grease a 9x13-inch baking pan. Rinse orange, grate off 1 tablespoon zest, and squeeze out juice, straining out seeds. Set aside.

2. Combine fresh cranberries, dried cranberries, ½ cup sugar, cranberry juice cocktail, Triple Sec, orange juice, and orange zest in a 2-quart saucepan. Bring to a boil over medium-high heat, reduce heat to medium, and cook, stirring occasionally, for 10 minutes, or until cranberries pop. Add apples, and cook, stirring occasionally, for an additional 10 minutes, or until apples begin to soften.

3. Combine remaining sugar, rice flour, potato starch, tapioca flour, baking powder, xanthan gum, and salt in a mixing bowl. Whisk well. Combine eggs, cream, and sour cream in another mixing bowl, and whisk until smooth. Add flour mixture, and mix until well incorporated.

4. Form dough into 12 mounds and arrange them on top of fruit. Bake for 35 to 40 minutes, or until golden. Serve hot or at room temperature with sweetened whipped cream or ice cream on top, if using.

Note: The fruit mixture can be prepared up to 2 days in advance and refrigerated, tightly covered. Reheat it to a simmer, covered, over low heat, stirring occasionally.

Variations:
* *Substitute pears for the apples.*
* *Substitute dried tart cherries or dried blueberries for the dried cranberries.*

There has been a glut of cranberries on the market for several years, but they're usually only available in season and few manufacturers sell them frozen. It's easy to do yourself, though. In fact, just toss the bags you find around the holidays right into the freezer. You can rinse them after they're thawed.

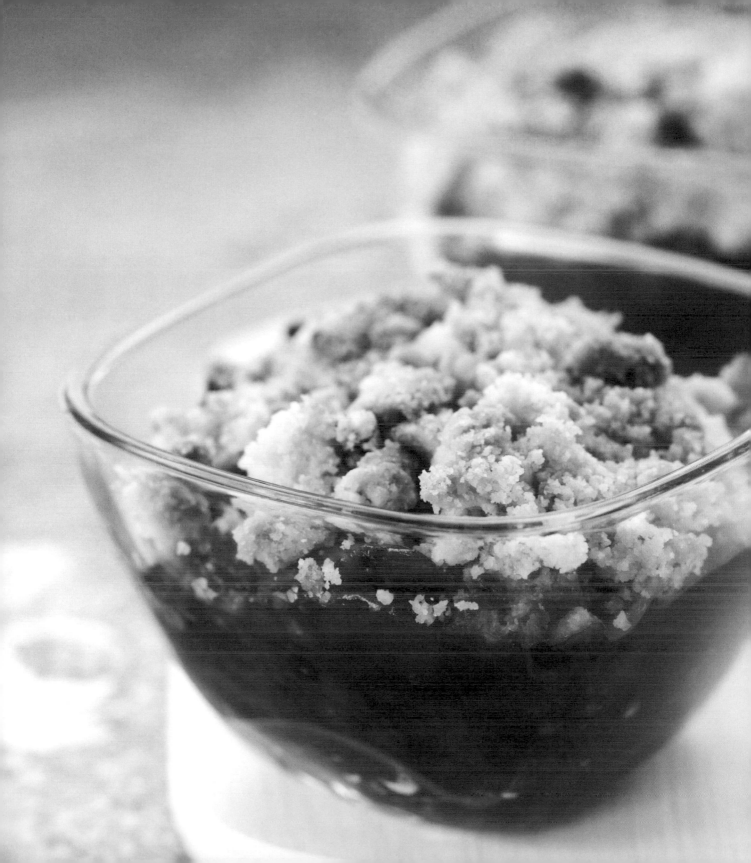

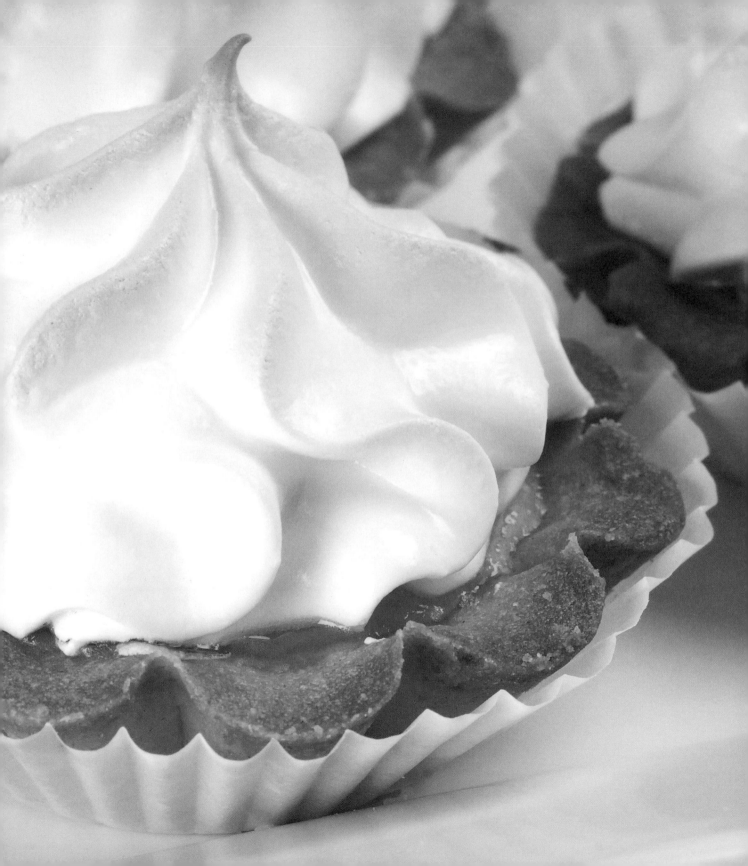

Pumpkin Pecan Cheesecake Bites

Miniature cheesecake bites are a great addition to any dessert buffet. These moist and rich treats are flavored like a traditional pumpkin pie, with a crust made from crunchy pecans.

Yield: Makes 2 dozen

Active time: 20 minutes

Start to finish: 6 hours, including time to chill

1½ cups toasted pecans

3 tablespoons firmly packed light brown sugar

3 tablespoons unsalted butter, melted

1¼ teaspoons ground cinnamon, divided

3 (8-ounce) packages cream cheese, softened

1¼ cups granulated sugar

4 large eggs

1 15-ounce can pure pumpkin

½ cup half-and-half

2 tablespoons brown rice flour

1 teaspoon pure vanilla extract

¾ teaspoon ground ginger

¼ teaspoon salt

Sweetened whipped cream

1. Preheat the oven to 350°F. Line a 9x13-inch pan with heavy-duty aluminum foil, with the foil extending up 3 inches on the short sides of the pan. Grease the foil heavily.

2. Combine pecans, light brown sugar, melted butter, and ¼ teaspoon cinnamon in a food processor fitted with the steel blade. Process until mixture forms a ball. Press mixture into the bottom of the pan, and bake for 15 minutes, or until golden. Cool crust completely.

3. Combine cream cheese and sugar in a mixing bowl, and beat until smooth. Add eggs 1 at a time, and then add pumpkin, half-and-half, rice flour, vanilla, ginger, salt, and remaining cinnamon. Pour batter over the baked crust.

4. Place the pan inside a larger roasting pan in the oven. Pour enough boiling water into the roasting pan to come halfway up sides of cheesecake. Bake for 1 hour. Turn off the oven and allow cake to sit in the water bath for 1 hour more. Cool cake to room temperature on a wire rack, and then refrigerate until well chilled.

5. Remove cake from the pan by pulling up on the sides of the foil. Cut out circles using a 2-inch round biscuit cutter. Top each circle with a swirl of sweetened whipped cream.

Note: The cheesecake can be made up to 2 days in advance and refrigerated. Do not add the whipped cream until just prior to serving.

Variation:
* *Substitute hazelnuts, walnuts, or almonds for the pecans.*

> **Be careful when shopping for pumpkin.** Right next to the cans of solid-pack pumpkin, which is a great convenience because it's pure pumpkin that is cooked and pureed, are cans of pumpkin pie filling. This has sugar, spices, evaporated milk, and usually gluten-containing wheat flour added.

Warm Chocolate Tortes

These upside-down cupcakes have a center of molten chocolate, and they're popular the world over. They're an elegant way to end a holiday dinner, or they're delicious enough to make any dinner into a holiday.

Yield: 6 servings

Active time: 20 minutes

Start to finish: 40 minutes

5 ounces high-quality bittersweet chocolate, chopped, divided

2 tablespoons heavy cream

1 tablespoon rum or fruit-flavored liqueur

3 tablespoons brown rice flour

2 tablespoons cornstarch

½ teaspoon xanthan gum

¼ teaspoon salt

5 tablespoons unsalted butter, sliced

2 large eggs

1 large egg yolk

¼ cup granulated sugar

Sweetened whipped cream or ice cream for serving (optional)

1. Melt 2 ounces of chocolate, cream, and rum in a small microwave-safe dish. Stir well and refrigerate to harden. Form the chocolate into 6 balls and refrigerate until ready to use.

2. Preheat the oven to 350°F. Grease six cups of a standard muffin pan.

3. Combine rice flour, cornstarch, xanthan gum, and salt in a mixing bowl. Whisk well.

4. Melt remaining chocolate with butter and allow to cool. Place the eggs, egg yolk, and sugar in a medium mixing bowl. Beat with an electric mixer at medium and then high speed until very thick and triple in volume. Fold cooled chocolate into eggs, then fold in rice flour mixture.

5. Divide batter among the muffin tins and push a chocolate ball into the center of each tin. Bake tortes for 10 to 12 minutes, or until sides are set. Remove the pan from the oven and invert onto a baking sheet. Serve immediately, with whipped cream or ice cream, if using.

Note: The tortes can be prepared up to 2 hours before baking them. However, they must bake just prior to serving.

Variation:
* *Substitute 1 tablespoon instant espresso powder dissolved in 1 tablespoon water for the rum.*

> **Like fine wine, dark chocolate actually improves with age. Store it tightly wrapped in a cool place. Even if the chocolate has developed a gray "bloom" from being stored at too high a temperature, it is still fine to use for cooking.**

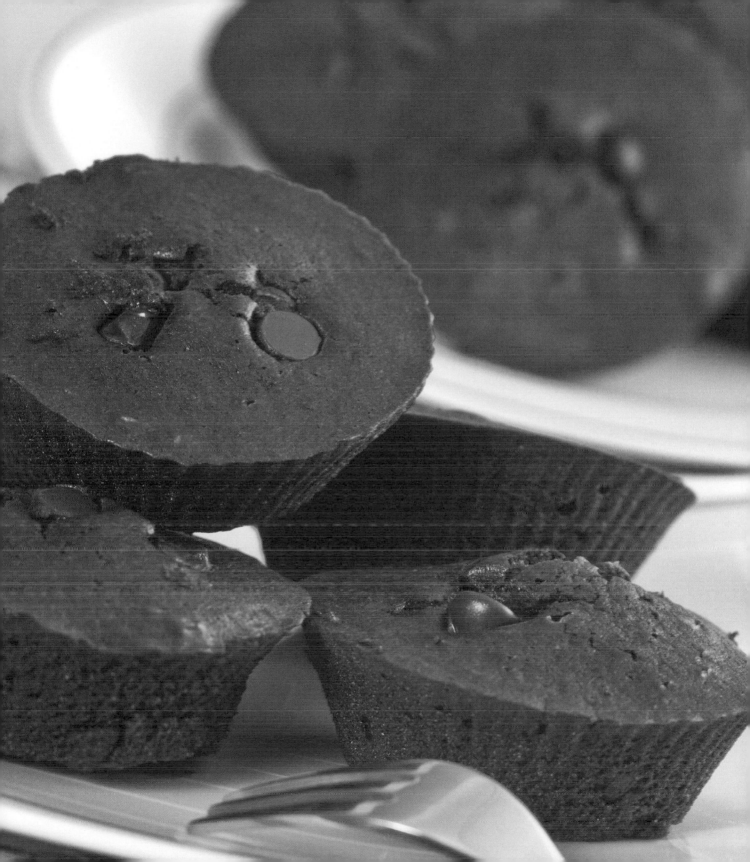

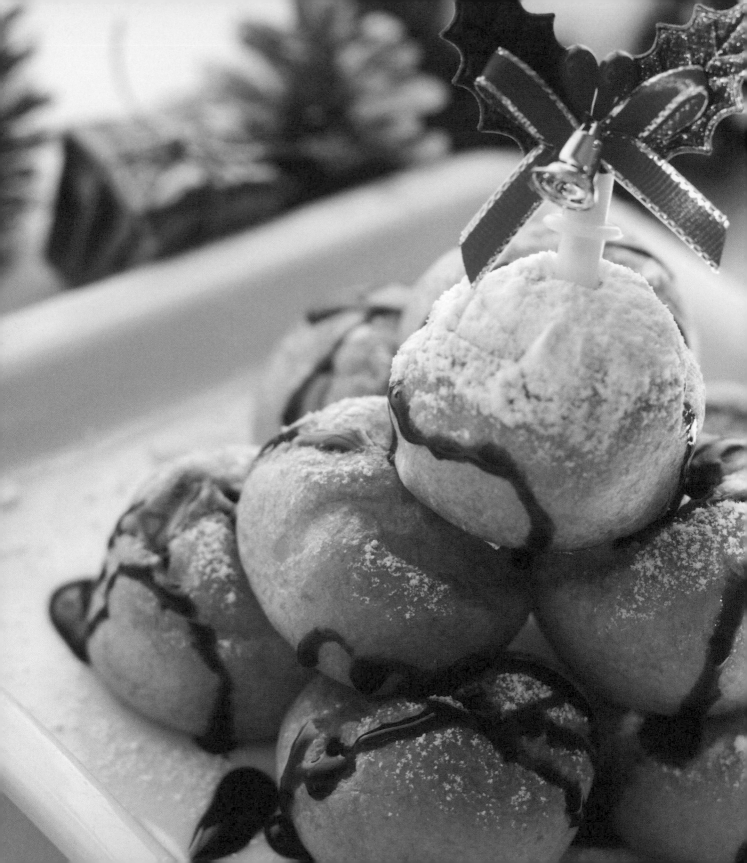

Profiteroles

These baby cream puffs can be filled with pastry cream or ice cream and topped with a sauce or a glaze of chocolate.

Yield: 3 dozen

Active time: 20 minutes

Start to finish: 1 hour

½ cup white rice flour

¼ cup potato starch

2 tablespoons tapioca flour

½ teaspoon xanthan gum

½ teaspoon salt

6 tablespoons (¾ stick) unsalted butter

2 teaspoons granulated sugar

½ teaspoon kosher salt

¼ teaspoon pure vanilla extract

5 large eggs, divided

1 to 1½ pints ice cream, softened

1. Preheat the oven to 425°F, and line two baking sheets with parchment paper or silicone baking mats.

2. Combine rice flour, potato starch, tapioca flour, xanthan gum, and salt in a bowl, and whisk well. Combine butter, sugar, salt, vanilla, and 1 cup of water in a saucepan, and bring to a boil over medium-high heat, stirring occasionally. Remove the pan from the heat, and add flour mixture all at once. Using a wooden paddle or wide wooden spoon, beat the flour into the liquid until it is smooth.

3. Place the saucepan over high heat and beat mixture constantly for 1 to 2 minutes, or until it forms a mass that leaves the sides of the pan and begins to film the bottom of the pot.

4. Transfer mixture to a food processor fitted with the steel blade. Add 4 of the eggs, 1 at a time, beating well between each addition and scraping the sides of the work bowl between each addition. (This can also be done by hand, but it takes a long time to beat it until the eggs are incorporated.)

5. Scrape dough into a pastry bag fitted with a ½-inch round nozzle. Pipe mounds 1-inch in diameter and ½-inch high onto the baking sheets, allowing 2 inches between the puffs.

6. Beat remaining egg with a pinch of salt, and brush only tops of the dough mounds with a small pastry brush or rub gently with a finger dipped in the egg wash. (Be careful not to drip egg wash onto the baking sheet or egg may prevent dough from puffing.)

7. Bake puffs for 20 to 25 minutes, or until golden brown and crusty to the touch. Remove the pans from the oven. Use the tip of a paring knife to cut a slit in the side of each puff to allow steam to escape. Turn off the oven, and place baked puffs back into the oven with the oven door ajar for 5 minutes. Remove puffs, and transfer to a wire rack to cool. To serve, split puffs with a serrated knife, and fill with ice cream.

Note: The puffs can be made up to 1 day in advance and kept at room temperature.

Variation:

✷ *To make 12 large cream puffs: Make the mounds of dough 2½ inches wide and 1 inch high. Or pipe the dough into lines of these dimensions for éclair shape. Bake at 425°F for 20 minutes, and then reduce the heat to 375°F and bake for an additional 10–15 minutes. Remove the pans from the oven, and split puffs using a serrated knife. Turn off the oven, and place baked puffs back into the oven with the oven door ajar for 10 minutes to finish crisping. Cool puffs in halves rather than whole, and pull out any dough from the center of the puffs that might be soggy.*

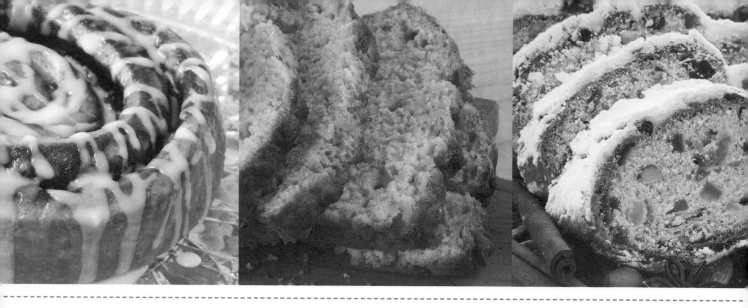

CHAPTER 4:

The Gluten-Free Breadbasket:

Quick Breads, Yeast Breads, Muffins, and Biscuits

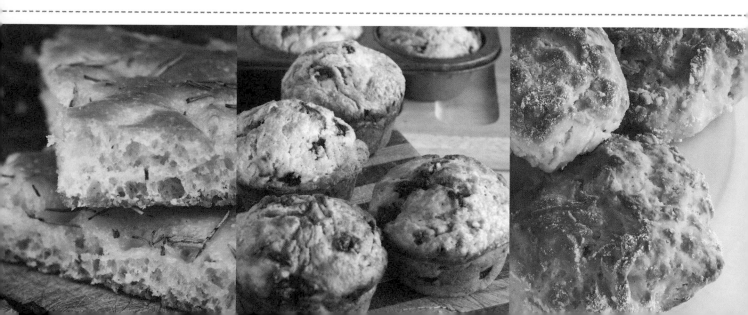

W aking up to the tantalizing aromas of butter melding with cinnamon in the morning, a bonus of sticky buns baking in the oven, is enough to make any day a holiday. And serving savory muffins as a side dish for Christmas dinner makes that meal more festive too.

Then there are specific breads from different cuisines associated with Christmas. These include two made with succulent dried fruit: Pannetone from Italy and Stollen from Germany. You'll find recipes for those in this chapter in their gluten-free versions too.

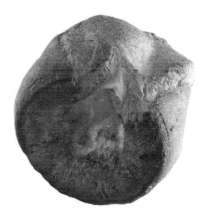

Yeasty Matters

If you don't make yeast-risen breads because you are intimidated by working with yeast, now is the time to take the plunge. The whole process could not be easier, and here's a primer on how to work with this live leavening agent.

All bread depends on the interaction of some sort of flour, liquid, and leavening agent. When the proteins in wheat flour combine with water, they form gluten. Gluten has both plasticity and elasticity. It will hold the carbon dioxide produced by the yeast and will not allow it to escape or break. It is this plasticity that allows bread to rise before it is baked, at which time the structure of the dough solidifies from the heat of the oven. You can create wonderful yeast breads without gluten, as you'll see when baking the recipes in this chapter. But instead of one ingredient—wheat flour—you'll be using formulations of various gluten-free products.

Yeast, unlike baking soda and baking powder, is an organic leavening agent, which means that it must be "alive" to be effective. Overly high temperatures can kill yeast; on the other hand, cold temperatures can inhibit the yeast's action. That is why dry yeast should be refrigerated. It will keep for several months.

To make sure your yeast is alive, you should start with a step called "proofing." Combine the yeast with warm liquid (110–115°F) and a small amount of rice flour or sugar. If the water is any hotter, it might kill the yeast. Either use a meat thermometer to take the temperature or make sure it feels warm but not hot on the underside of your wrist. Think of it as the baby bottle test.

Let the mixture rest at room temperature until a thick surface foam forms, which indicates that the yeast is alive and can be used. If there is no foam, the yeast is dead and should be discarded. After your proofing is successful, you are ready to make the dough.

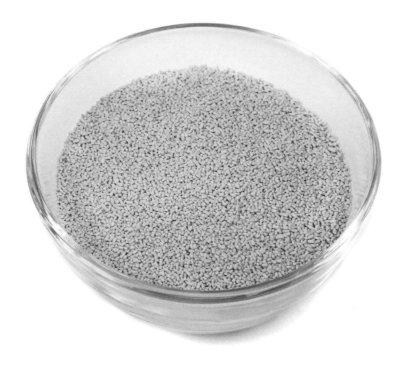

Chemical leavening is nothing new; Amelia Simmons used pearl ash in her book *American Cookery,* published in 1796. Because carbon dioxide is released at a faster rate through the acid-base reaction than through the fermentation process provided by living yeast, breads made with chemical leavening became known as "quick breads" more than a century ago.

The right temperature is necessary for dough to rise. There are some tricks to creating a warm enough temperature in a cold kitchen. Set a foil-covered electric heating pad on low, and put the bowl of dough on the foil; put the bowl in the dishwasher and set if for just the drying cycle; put the bowl in your gas oven to benefit from the warmth from the pilot light; put the bowl in any cold oven over a large pan of boiling-hot water.

Marvelous Muffins and Easy Quick Breads

Muffins and quick breads are being discussed together because the batters are identical in preparation and they're interchangeable; the only difference is the amount of time and at what temperature they are baked.

Quick breads are so named since they are made with a chemical leavening agent, thus eliminating the time spent waiting for yeast bread dough to rise. Quick breads can be served as an alternative not only to yeast-raised breads but also in place of potatoes or rice as a base for stews or other braised dishes. Leftover muffins can be used to create a bread pudding, and leftover quick bread can be turned into a wonderful French toast or stuffing (by first toasting the cubes).

Convertible Forms

The difference between muffins and quick breads is the amount of time needed to bake them through and at what temperature they should be baked. Use this chart for guidance if you want to convert one form to another.

Baked Good	Time	Temperature
Standard Muffins	18–22 minutes	400°F
Oversized Muffins	20–25 minutes	375°F
Quick Breads	45 minutes to 1 hour	350°F

Pannetone

It wouldn't be Christmas in many Italian households without this vertical yeast bread studded with candied fruit. It makes a very dramatic presentation, and the flavor is delicious.

Yield: Makes 3 loaves

Active Time: 30 minutes

Start to finish: 4½ hours

1 cup brown rice flour

1 cup tapioca flour

3¾ cups cornstarch

2 tablespoons xanthan gum

2 (¼-ounce) packages active dry yeast

1 teaspoon salt

1 cup golden raisins

½ cup sweet Marsala

2 cups warm whole milk (110–115°F)

1 cup honey

4 large eggs, at room temperature

1 cup (2 sticks) unsalted butter, melted and cooled

2 teaspoons pure vanilla extract

1½ cups chopped candied fruit

1 large egg yolk

Note: Have three empty coffee cans handy.

1. Combine brown rice flour, tapioca flour, cornstarch, xanthan gum, yeast, and salt in a mixing bowl. Whisk well. Combine raisins and Marsala in a small microwave-safe bowl. Microwave on High (100 percent power) for 40 seconds.

2. Combine milk, honey, eggs, butter, and vanilla in the mixing bowl of a standard mixer fitted with the paddle attachment. Beat at medium speed for 1 minute. Reduce the speed to low, and add flour mixture. Beat at low speed for 2 minutes. Drain raisins, discarding any Marsala remaining. Add raisins and candied fruit to dough.

3. Cover the bowl loosely with a sheet of plastic wrap, and place it in a warm spot for 1–2 hours, or until dough is doubled in bulk.

4. Grease 3 (1-pound) empty coffee cans. Divide dough into 3 parts, and place each in a prepared can. Cover loosely with plastic wrap, and allow to rise for 1 hour.

5. While dough rises, preheat the oven to 350°F. Mix egg yolk with 2 tablespoons water, and brush tops of loaves with mixture. Bake loaves for 45–50 minutes, or until deep brown and firm. Allow to cool for 5 minutes, then turn onto a wire rack to cool completely.

Note: The loaves can be baked up to 3 days in advance and refrigerated, tightly covered with plastic wrap. Baked loaves can also be frozen for up to 2 months.

Variations:
* *Substitute brandy or a fruit liqueur for the Marsala.*
* *Substitute pure almond extract for the vanilla extract, soak the raisins in amaretto or other almond-flavored liqueur, and substitute ½ cup chopped toasted almonds for ½ cup of the candied fruit.*

Marsala, like Sherry and Port, is a fortified wine. It is usually between 16 and 18 percent alcohol. It made with three different varietals of Italian grapes, and it became very popular in the mid-eighteenth century in England, which boosted domestic production in Italy.

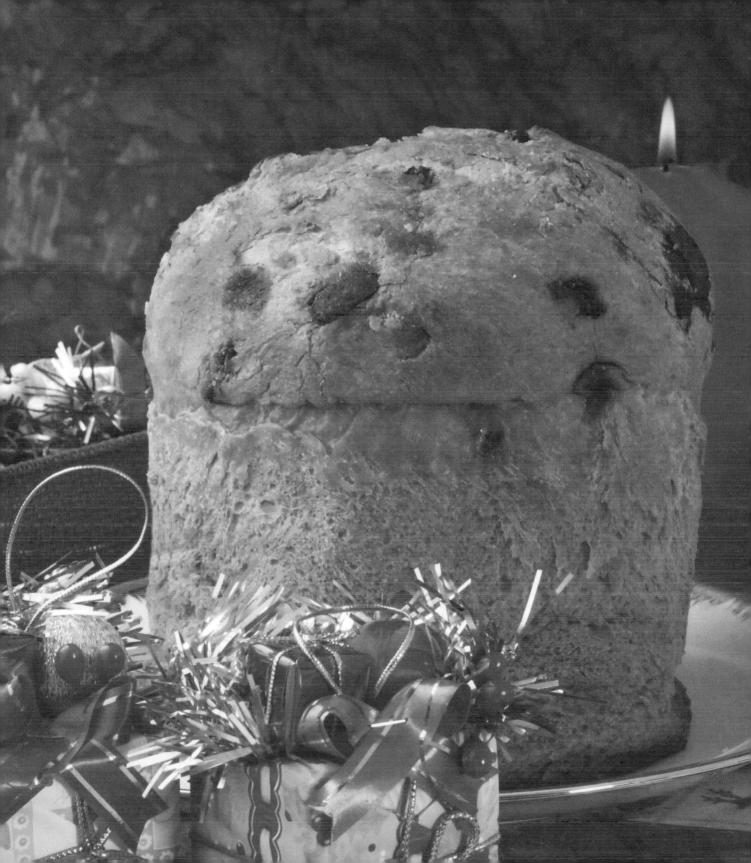

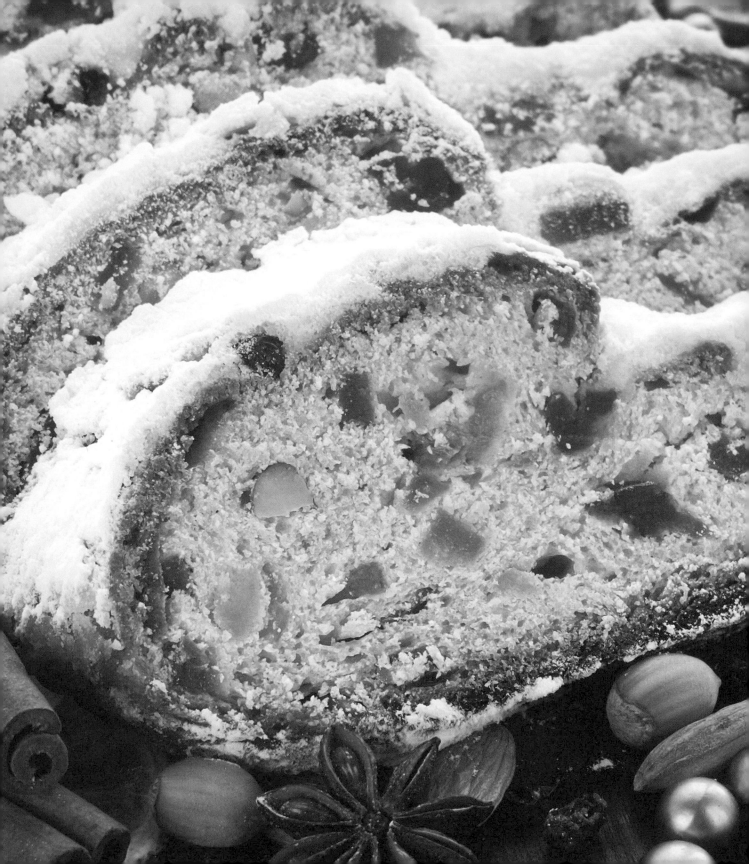

Stollen

Christmas breads are common in many European cuisines, and this one is from Germany. The bread is so laden with dried and candied fruit that the dough merely binds it together.

Yield: Makes 2 loaves

Active time: 30 minutes

Start to finish: 4½ hours plus an overnight for the fruit to macerate

1 cup black raisins

1 cup golden raisins

½ cup dried cherries

½ cup dried cranberries

½ cup rum

1 cup brown rice flour

1 cup tapioca flour

3¾ cups cornstarch

2 tablespoons xanthan gum

2 (¼-ounce) packages active dry yeast

1 teaspoon salt

1 teaspoon ground cinnamon

1 teaspoon freshly grated nutmeg

½ teaspoon ground cardamom

2 cups warm whole milk (110–115°F)

1 cup honey

4 large eggs, at room temperature

1 cup (2 sticks) unsalted butter, melted and cooled

1 tablespoon grated orange zest

½ teaspoon pure vanilla extract

1 cup sliced almonds

½ cup chopped crystallized ginger

1 cup Royal Icing (page 17)

Note: Be prepared to let the fruit macerate overnight.

1. Combine black raisins, golden raisins, dried cherries, dried cranberries, and rum in a mixing bowl. Stir well. Cover with plastic wrap and allow fruits to macerate overnight.

2. Preheat the oven to 350°F. Toast almonds on a baking sheet for 5–7 minutes, or until browned. Set aside. Turn off oven.

3. Combine brown rice flour, tapioca flour, cornstarch, xanthan gum, yeast, salt, cinnamon, nutmeg, and cardamom in a mixing bowl. Whisk well.

4. Combine milk, honey, eggs, butter, orange zest, and vanilla in the mixing bowl of a standard mixer fitted with the paddle attachment. Beat at medium speed for 1 minute. Reduce the speed to low, and add flour mixture. Beat at low speed for 2 minutes. Add macerated fruit, almonds, and crystallized ginger. Beat for 1 minute.

5. Cover the bowl loosely with a sheet of plastic wrap, and place it in a warm spot for 1–2 hours, or until dough is doubled in bulk.

6. Line a baking sheet with parchment paper or silicone baking mats. Divide dough in half, and form each into an oval 8 inches long. Cover loaves lightly with a tea towel, and allow them to rise for 1 hour, or until very puffy.

7. While loaves rise, preheat the oven to 350°F. Bake loaves for 1 hour, or until firm and brown. Cool on the pan for 10 minutes, then transfer loaves to a wire rack to cool completely. When loaves are cool, frost tops with Royal Icing.

Note: The loaves can be baked up to 3 days in advance and kept at room temperature, tightly covered.

Variation:

* *Substitute bourbon or brandy for the rum.*

Popovers

Popovers are a light and crusty treat that make a meal really special. But they have be baked right before serving, so make sure your oven will be cleared from all other dishes.

Yield: 1 dozen

Active time: 10 minutes

Start to finish: 50 minutes

½ cup white rice flour

⅓ cup potato starch

¼ cup tapioca flour

½ teaspoon salt

¼ teaspoon xanthan gum

1¼ cups whole milk, slightly warm

4 large eggs

3 tablespoons unsalted butter, melted and cooled

1. Preheat the oven to 400ºF. Grease a 12-cup popover pan or muffin pan.

2. Combine rice flour, potato starch, tapioca flour, salt, and xanthan gum in a mixing bowl. Whisk well.

3. Combine milk, eggs, and butter in a blender or food processor fitted with the steel blade. Blend until smooth. Add flour mixture, and blend until smooth.

4. Spoon batter into the prepared cups with a ladle, filling each ⅔ full. Bake for 25 minutes. Reduce the oven temperature to 350ºF, and bake for an additional 10 minutes, or until the tops are browned. Remove the pan from the oven, and allow popovers to sit for 3 minutes, then serve.

Note: The batter can be made up to 4 hours in advance and kept at room temperature. Blend it again to distribute the ingredients before filling the cups.

Variations:
* *Add 2 teaspoons grated lemon zest and 1 tablespoon finely chopped fresh rosemary to the batter.*
* *Add 1 tablespoon grated orange zest, 1 tablespoon granulated sugar, and ½ teaspoon ground ginger to the batter.*
* *Yorkshire pudding is just popovers baked in the pan in which standing rib roast was baked. You can use this same recipe.*

> **What makes popovers rise in the oven is the steam created in the batter because they are cooked at a high temperature. The steam pushes up the structure of the eggs, and then the combination of flours and starches solidifies along with the eggs.**

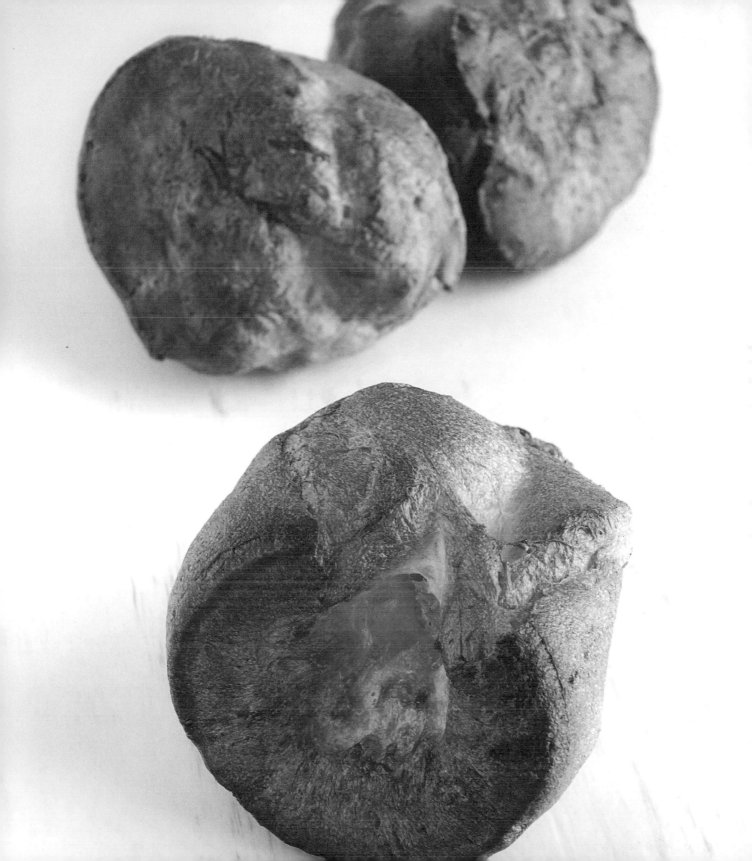

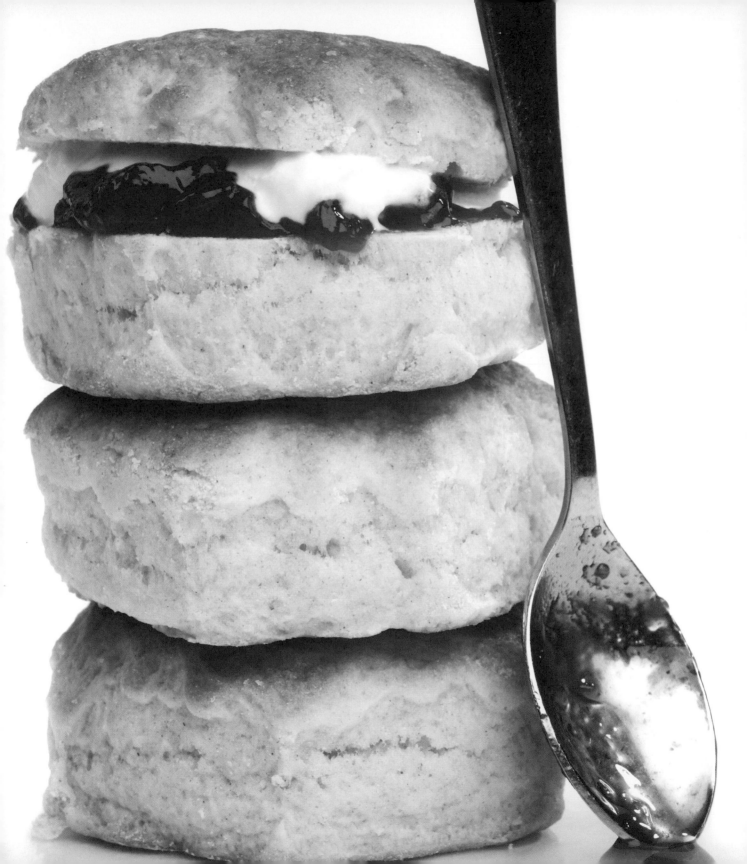

Scones

Scones are the British equivalent of biscuits, and they're served as part of a traditional afternoon tea. They are also wonderfully rich breads to serve at a holiday brunch.

Yield: 1 dozen

Active time: 15 minutes

Start to finish: 35 minutes

1 cup white rice flour

⅔ cup potato starch

⅔ cup tapioca flour

¼ cup granulated sugar

1 tablespoon gluten-free baking powder

½ teaspoon xanthan gum

½ teaspoon salt

2 large eggs, lightly beaten

¾ cup heavy cream

¼ cup sour cream

1 large egg yolk, lightly beaten

2 tablespoons whole milk

1. Preheat the oven to 400°F. Line a baking sheet with parchment paper or a silicone baking mat.

2. Combine rice flour, potato starch, tapioca flour, sugar, baking powder, xanthan gum, and salt in a mixing bowl. Whisk well.

3. Combine eggs, cream, and sour cream in another mixing bowl, and whisk until smooth. Add flour mixture, and mix until well incorporated.

4. Form dough into 12 mounds on the baking sheet about 1½ inches high. Combine egg yolk and milk in a small cup. Brush tops of biscuits with egg wash.

5. Bake scones for 14–17 minutes, or until browned. Serve immediately.

Note: The scones can be made up to 1 day in advance and kept at room temperature, tightly covered. Reheat them in a 300°F oven, covered with foil, for 5–7 minutes.

Variations:
* *Add ½ cup dried currants or dried cranberries to the dough.*
* *Add 1 tablespoon grated orange zest and 1 teaspoon grated lemon zest to the dough.*
* *Substitute firmly packed dark brown sugar for the granulated sugar.*

Scones are traditionally served in England at afternoon tea with some sort of fruit preserves and clotted cream. This high-fat, high-flavor thick cream is easy to replicate in your own kitchen. Combine 4 ounces mascarpone with 1 cup heavy whipping cream. Add a few tablespoons of sugar if you care to make it slightly sweet. That's it. Enjoy!

Old-Fashioned Southern Biscuits

Biscuits are to the Southern states what a baguette is to France; it's the form of bread eaten at just about every meal. These gluten-free biscuits are incredibly light and tender, and they're delicious with butter and jam or with sausage gravy.

Yield: 1 dozen

Active time: 15 minutes

Start to finish: 30 minutes

1 cup white rice flour

¾ cup potato starch

¾ cup tapioca flour

2 tablespoons gluten-free baking powder

2 tablespoons granulated sugar

1 tablespoon xanthan gum

½ teaspoon salt

2 large eggs, lightly beaten

1½ cups buttermilk

½ cup (1 stick) unsalted butter, melted

1 large egg yolk, lightly beaten

2 tablespoons whole milk

1. Preheat the oven to 375°F. Line a baking sheet with parchment paper or a silicone baking mat.

2. Combine rice flour, potato starch, tapioca flour, baking powder, sugar, xanthan gum, and salt in a mixing bowl. Whisk well.

3. Combine eggs, buttermilk, and butter in another mixing bowl, and whisk until smooth. Add flour mixture, and mix until well incorporated.

4. Form dough into 12 mounds about 2½ inches wide. Combine egg yolk and milk in a small cup. Brush tops of biscuits with egg wash.

5. Bake biscuits for 12–15 minutes, or until browned. Serve immediately.

Note: The biscuits can be made up to 1 day in advance and kept at room temperature, tightly covered. Reheat them in a 300°F oven, covered with foil, for 5–7 minutes.

Variations:

* *Add ¼ cup canned chopped mild green chiles, drained, and ½ cup grated cheddar cheese.*
* *Combine ½ cup firmly packed dark brown sugar, ½ teaspoon ground cinnamon, and ½ cup finely chopped pecans. Pat the mixture on the tops of the biscuits before baking.*
* *Add 2 tablespoons chopped fresh herbs to the dough.*
* *Add ½ cup freshly grated Parmesan and 1 teaspoon Italian seasoning.*
* *Add ½ cup chopped scallions, white parts and 4 inches of green tops.*

The American meaning for biscuit was first noted by John Palmer in his *Journal of Travels in the United States of North America, and in Lower Canada,* (1818), and by 1828 Webster defined the confection as "a composition of flour and butter, made and baked in private families." Recipes for biscuits are found in every nineteenth-century cookbook, especially with reference to the cookery of the South.

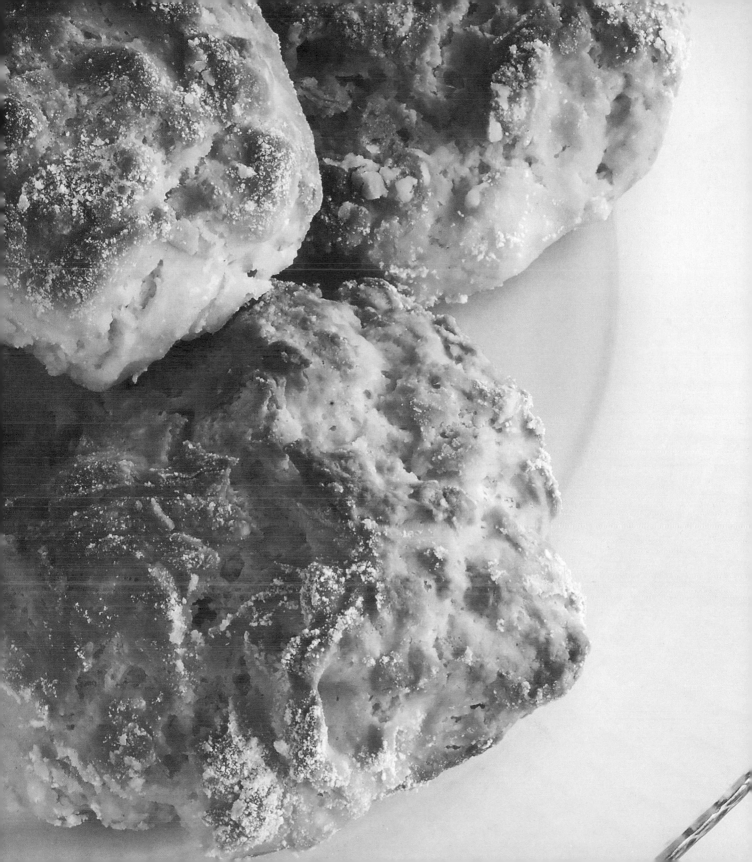

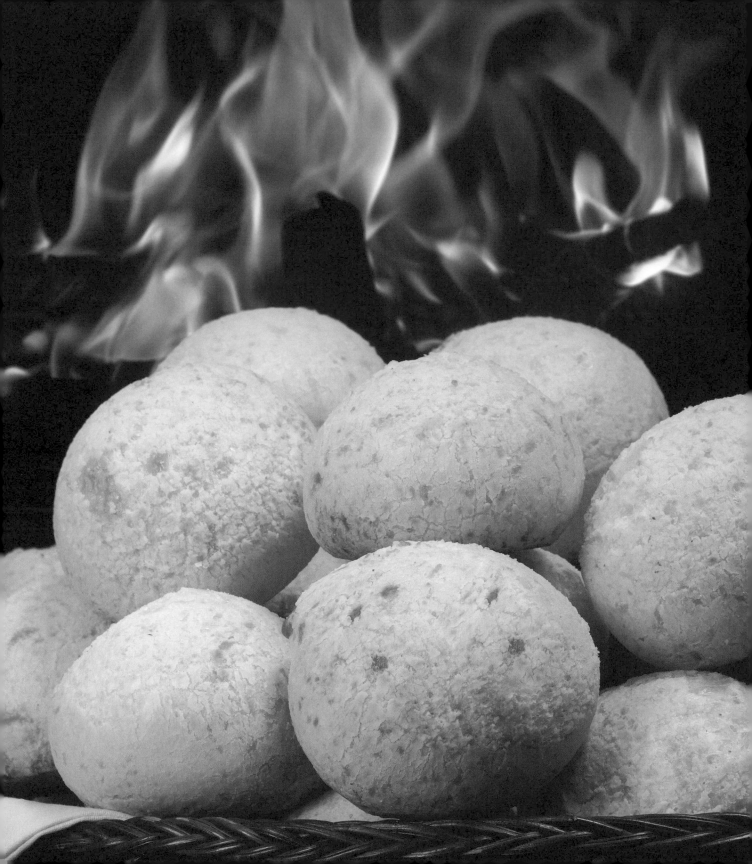

Brazilian Garlicky Cheese Rolls

These light and puffy rolls, called Pão de Queijo in Portuguese, are similar to Gougères (see page 117). They are a light and luscious addition to any meal.

Yield: 1½ dozen

Active time: 15 minutes

Start to finish: 35 minutes

½ cup (1 stick) unsalted butter, sliced

½ cup whole milk

½ teaspoon salt

2 garlic cloves, minced

2 cups tapioca flour

2 large eggs

⅔ cup freshly grated Parmesan cheese

Freshly ground black pepper to taste

1. Preheat the oven to 375°F, and line two baking sheets with parchment paper or silicone baking mats.

2. Combine butter, milk, salt, and garlic in a small saucepan, and bring to a boil over medium-high heat, stirring occasionally. Remove the pan from the heat, and add tapioca flour mixture all at once. Using a wooden paddle or wide wooden spoon, beat dry ingredients into liquid until smooth. Then place the saucepan over high heat and beat mixture constantly for 1–2 minutes, or until it forms a mass that leaves the sides of the pan and begins to film the bottom of the pot.

3. Transfer mixture to a food processor fitted with the steel blade. Add eggs, 1 at a time, beating well between each addition and scraping the sides of the work bowl between each addition. Then add cheese and pepper, and mix well again.

4. Using a soupspoon dipped in cold water, form dough into 2-tablespoon mounds on the baking sheets, allowing 2 inches between puffs.

5. Bake rolls for 18–20 minutes, or lightly browned. Serve immediately.

Note: The rolls can be prepared up to 6 hours in advance and kept at room temperature. Reheat the rolls in a microwave oven. Microwave on High (100 percent power) in 20-second intervals until hot.

Variations:
* *Substitute Romano or Asiago for the Parmesan.*
* *Add ¼ cup finely chopped cooked bacon or ham to the dough.*
* *Add 2 tablespoons chopped fresh basil and 2 tablespoons finely chopped sun-dried tomatoes to the dough.*

> **The way you treat garlic determines the intensity of its flavor. Pushing the cloves through a garlic press is the way to extract the most punch. Mincing the cloves once they're peeled produces a milder flavor.**

Basic Focaccia

Focaccia (pronounced foe-KAH-cha) is one of the world's great nibble foods. It contains a fair amount of oil, so additional oil or butter isn't necessary to enjoy it, and it's flat so it's perfect for splitting to encase the filling for a sandwich. It's great on holiday buffets too.

Yield: 1 loaf (11x17 inches)

Active time: 20 minutes

Start to finish: 3½ hours

3 (¼-ounce) packages active dry yeast

2¼ cups warm water (110–115°F)

1 tablespoon granulated sugar

2½ cups brown rice flour, divided

1½ cups tapioca flour

2 cups soy flour

1 cup millet flour

2½ teaspoon xanthan gum

½ cup olive oil, divided

1 tablespoon kosher salt

Coarse salt and freshly ground black for sprinkling

1. Combine the yeast, water, sugar, and ¼ cup brown rice flour in the mixing bowl of a standard mixer, and whisk well to dissolve yeast. Set aside for 5 minutes, or until mixture begins to become foamy.

2. Combine remaining brown rice flour, tapioca flour, soy flour, millet flour, and xanthan gum in a mixing bowl. Whisk well.

3. Place the paddle attachment on the mixer. Add ⅓ cup oil, flour mixture, and salt. Beat a low speed until flour is incorporated to form a soft dough.

4. Place the dough hook on the mixer, and knead dough at medium speed for 2 minutes. Raise the speed to high, and knead for an additional 3–4 minutes, or until dough forms a soft ball and is springy. (If kneading by hand, it will take about 10–12 minutes.) Oil a mixing bowl, and add dough, turning it to make sure top is oiled. Cover the bowl loosely with a sheet of plastic wrap, and place it in a warm spot for 1–2 hours, or until dough is doubled in bulk.

5. Preheat the oven to 450°F, and oil a rimmed 11x17-inch baking sheet. Gently press dough into the prepared pan; allow dough to rest for 5 minutes if it is difficult to work with. Cover the pan with a sheet of oiled plastic wrap, and let rise in a warm place until doubled in bulk, about 30 minutes.

6. Make indentations in dough at 1-inch intervals with oiled fingertips. Drizzle top with remaining oil, and sprinkle it with coarse salt and pepper, or use one of the toppings listed in the Variations. Bake in the lower third of oven for 25–30 minutes, or until deep golden on top and pale golden on bottom. Transfer the bread to a wire cooling rack and serve warm or at room temperature.

Note: Bake up to 2 days in advance and keep at room temperature, tightly covered in plastic wrap.

Variations:
* ***Parmesan Olive Focaccia:*** *Sprinkle the top with ¾ cup freshly grated Parmesan cheese, and dot it with chopped olives.*
* ***Herb Focaccia:*** *Sprinkle the top with ½ cup of chopped fresh herbs, such as rosemary, basil, or oregano, or some combination.*
* ***Garlic Focaccia:*** *Soak four garlic cloves, peeled and minced, in the olive oil for 2 hours before making the dough. Either strain and discard garlic, or use it if you really like things garlicky.*

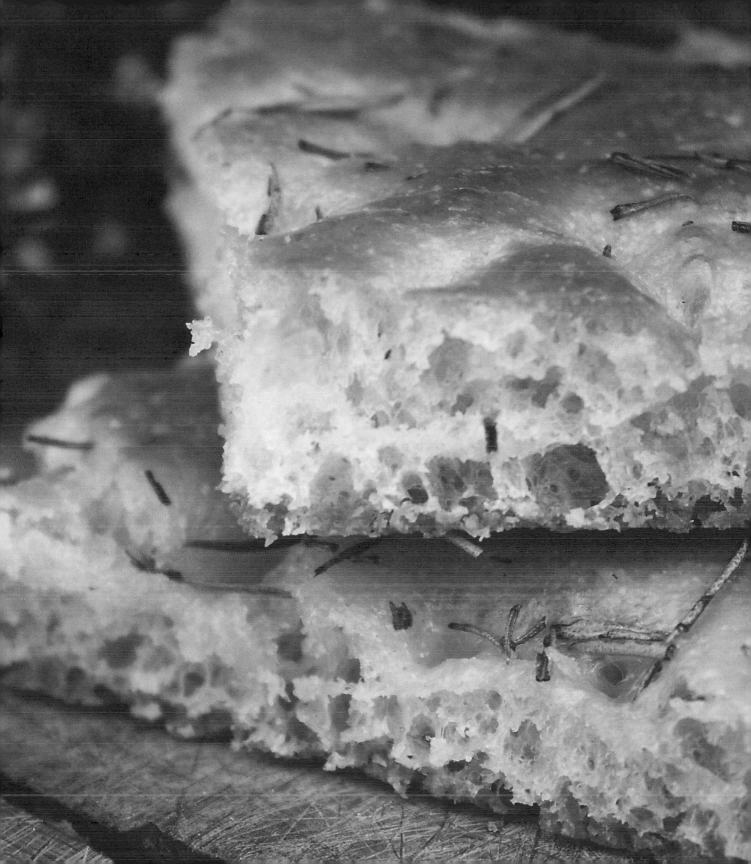

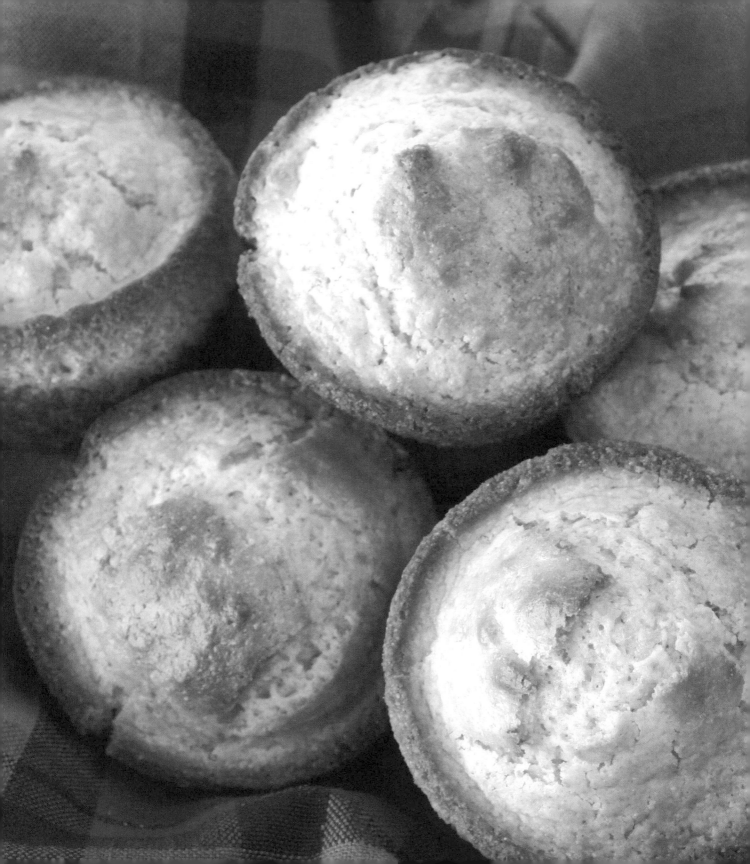

Cornmeal Cheese Muffins

Savory muffins are wonderful both at breakfast and as a dinner bread, and I like the combination of corn with the flavorful cheese. You can also toast up slices and spread it with cream cheese as an hors d'oeuvre.

Yield: 12 muffins

Active time: 10 minutes

Start to finish: 30 minutes

½ cup brown rice flour

⅓ cup potato starch

3 tablespoons tapioca flour

1 cup yellow gluten-free cornmeal

1 tablespoon gluten-free baking powder

1 tablespoon granulated sugar

½ teaspoon salt

½ teaspoon baking soda

⅛ teaspoon xanthan gum

1 cup buttermilk, shaken well

1 large egg

5 tablespoons unsalted butter, melted

1 cup grated cheddar cheese, divided

1. Preheat the oven to 400°F, and grease a 12-cup muffin pan; you can also use paper liners and spray the top of the pan with vegetable oil spray.

2. Combine rice flour, potato starch, tapioca flour, cornmeal, baking powder, sugar, salt, baking soda, and xanthan gum in a large mixing bowl, and whisk well. Add buttermilk, egg, butter, and ⅔ cup cheese. Stir gently to wet flour, but do not whisk until smooth; batter should be lumpy. Fill each prepared cup ⅔ full, and sprinkle with remaining cheese.

3. Bake muffins for 18–20 minutes, or until a toothpick inserted in the center comes out clean. Place muffin pan on a cooling rack for 10 minutes, then serve—either hot or at room temperature.

Variations:
* *Substitute jalapeño Jack for the cheddar cheese for a spicy, Southwestern muffin, and add ¼ teaspoon cayenne to the batter.*
* *Add ¾ cup crumbled cooked bacon and ½ cup finely chopped scallions to the batter.*
* *Add 1 tablespoon Italian seasoning and 1 garlic clove, peeled and pushed through a garlic press to the batter.*

Vegetable oil spray is a wonderful way to keep foods like cheese from becoming permanently bonded to your pans, but it also has a tendency to coat the counters. Open your dishwasher, and place the pan to be coated on the open door before you spray it. That keeps the counters clean, and any excess spray washes away the next time you use the dishwasher.

Parmesan Herb Muffins

Savory muffins are an alternative to breads on your dinner table, and because no yeast is used they can be on the table quickly. These go very well with a simple entrée like roast chicken or grilled fish.

Yield: 12 muffins

Active time: 10 minutes

Start to finish: 30 minutes

¾ cup white rice flour

½ cup potato starch

¼ cup tapioca flour

2 teaspoons gluten-free baking powder

2 teaspoons Italian seasoning

½ teaspoon baking soda

½ teaspoon xanthan gum

½ teaspoon salt

Freshly ground black pepper to taste

¾ cup whole milk

2 large eggs, beaten

½ cup olive oil

3 tablespoons chopped fresh parsley

1 cup freshly grated Parmesan cheese, divided

2 garlic cloves, minced

1. Preheat the oven to 400°F, and grease a 12-cup muffin pan; you can also use paper liners and spray the top of the pan with vegetable oil spray.

2. Combine rice flour, potato starch, tapioca flour, baking powder, Italian seasoning, baking soda, xanthan gum, salt, and pepper in a large mixing bowl, and whisk well. Add milk, eggs, oil, parsley, ⅔ cup cheese, and garlic. Stir gently to wet flour, but do not whisk until smooth; batter should be lumpy. Fill each prepared cup ⅔ full, and sprinkle with remaining cheese.

3. Bake muffins for 18–20 minutes, or until a toothpick inserted in the center comes out clean. Place muffin pan on a cooling rack for 10 minutes, then serve—either hot or at room temperature.

Variations:

✳ *Add ½ cup sun-dried tomatoes packed in olive oil, drained and chopped. Use the olive oil from the tomatoes as part of the oil for the recipe.*

✳ *Substitute dried oregano for the Italian seasoning, and add 1 tablespoon grated lemon zest.*

A display rack with pretty glass bottles over the stove is about the worst place to put dried herbs and spices because both heat and light are foes of these foods. Keep them in a cool, dark place to preserve their potency. The best test for freshness and potency is to smell the contents. If you don't smell a strong aroma, you need a new bottle.

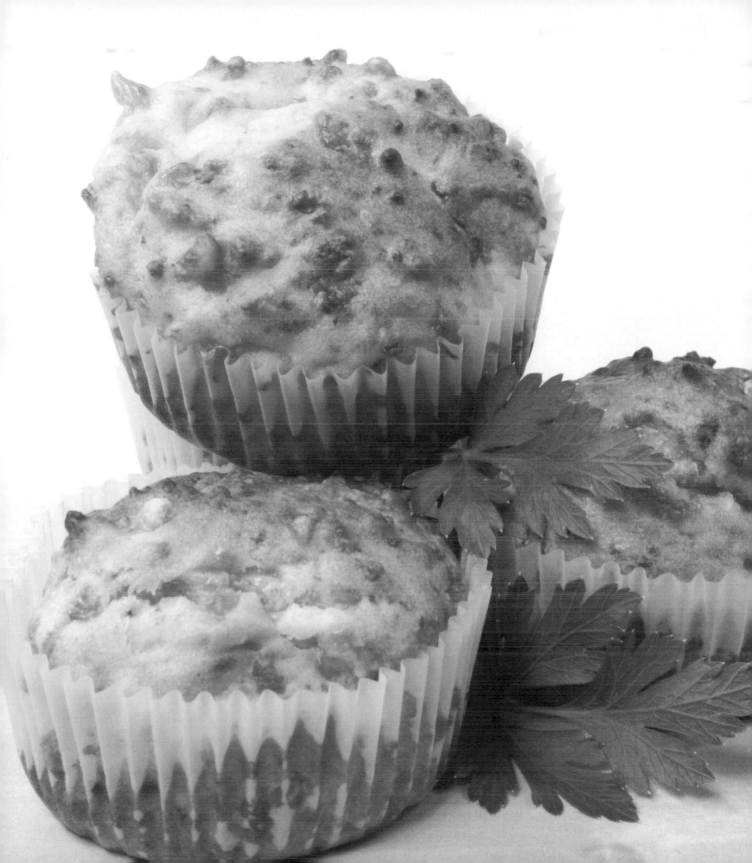

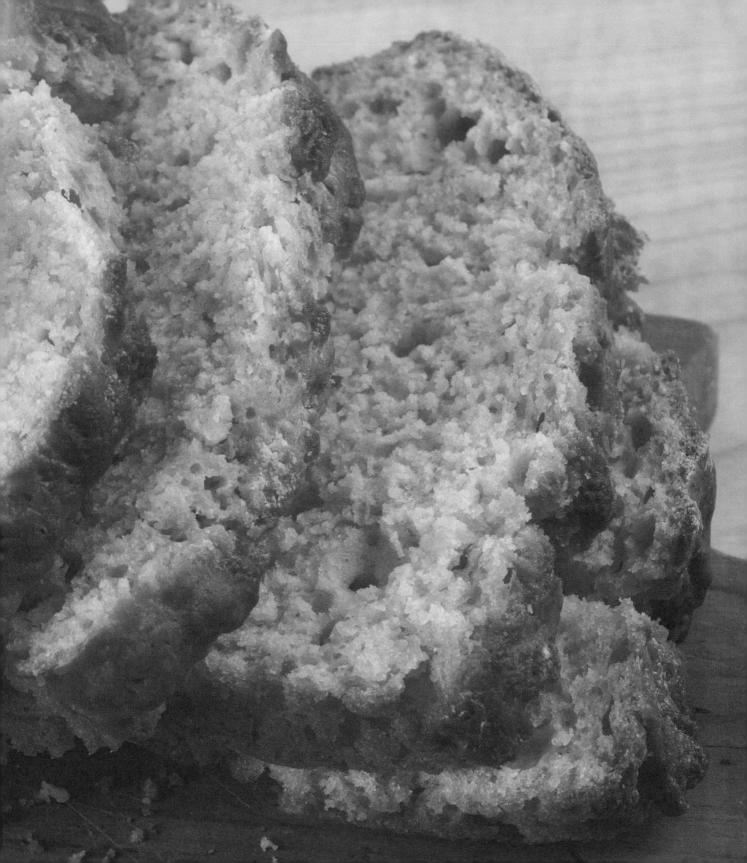

Beer Bread

I love beer bread because it has the same yeasty aroma and flavor as a rustic yeast bread, but it's so easy to make. In addition to serving it at dinner, I use it in place of sandwich bread.

Yield: 1 loaf

Active time: 10 minutes

Start to finish: 50 minutes

3½ cups all-purpose flour

1 teaspoon baking powder

1teaspoon xanthan gum

½ teaspoon salt

½ teaspoon baking soda

1 large egg, lightly beaten

1 (12-ounce) can gluten-free lager beer

1. Preheat the oven to 350°F, and grease a 9x5x3-inch loaf pan.

2. Combine flour, baking powder, xanthan gum, salt, and baking soda in a large mixing bowl, and whisk well. Add egg and beer, and stir until batter is just combined; batter should be lumpy. Scrape batter in the prepared pan.

3. Bake bread for 40–45 minutes, or until a toothpick inserted in the center comes out clean. Place pan on a cooling rack for 5 minutes, then turn bread out of the pan and serve—either hot or at room temperature.

Variations:
* *For a sweeter bread, add ½ cup granulated sugar to the batter.*
* *Add ½ cup chopped sun-dried tomatoes or ½ cup chopped oil-cured black olives, or ¼ cup of each to the batter.*
* *Add ½ cup chopped scallions, white parts and 3 inches of green tops, to the batter.*
* *Add ¼ cup chopped fresh dill to the batter.*

> Most beer is not gluten-free because it's made with malted barley; however, there is a large range of beer brands made with grains such as sorghum. The most widely available are Redbridge and Bard's Tale.

Irish Soda Bread

This hearty and rustic bread is one of the easiest to make, and it comes to the table looking pretty with a bright, shiny crust.

Yield: 2 (6-inch) loaves

Active time: 10 minutes

Start to finish: 50 minutes

2½ cups brown rice flour

⅔ cup potato starch

½ cup tapioca flour

2 tablespoons granulated sugar

1½ teaspoons baking soda

1 teaspoon xanthan gum

½ teaspoon salt

1¾ cups buttermilk, shaken well

2 tablespoons unsalted butter, melted

1. Preheat the oven to 375°F, grease a baking sheet and dust it with rice flour.

2. Combine rice flour, potato starch, tapioca flour, sugar, baking soda, xanthan gum, and salt in a large mixing bowl, and whisk well. Add buttermilk, and stir until batter is just combined; batter should be lumpy. Transfer dough to a well-floured surface, and knead with floured hands for 1 minute, or until dough is less sticky.

3. Divide dough in half, and pat each half into a 6-inch round on the prepared baking sheet. Cut an X that is ½-inch deep on top of each round, and brush tops with butter.

4. Bake bread for 35–40 minutes, or until tops are golden. Transfer loaves to a cooling rack with a wide spatula, and cool for at least 15 minutes.

Note: The bread can be served the day it is made, but it slices more easily if kept wrapped in plastic wrap at room temperature for 1 day, and up to 4 days.

Variations:
* *Add 1 cup raisins to dough, or 1 cup any chopped dried fruit such as dried apples or pitted dates.*
* *Add ½ cup chopped scallions, white parts and 3 inches of green tops.*
* *Add 2 tablespoons crushed caraway seeds or fennel seeds.*

> **Kneading is the process of working dough to make it pliable, so it will hold the gas bubbles from the leavening agent and expand when heated. Kneading is done with a pressing-folding-turning action. Press down into the dough with the heels of both hands, then push your hands away from your body. Fold the dough in half, and give it a quarter turn; then repeat the process.**

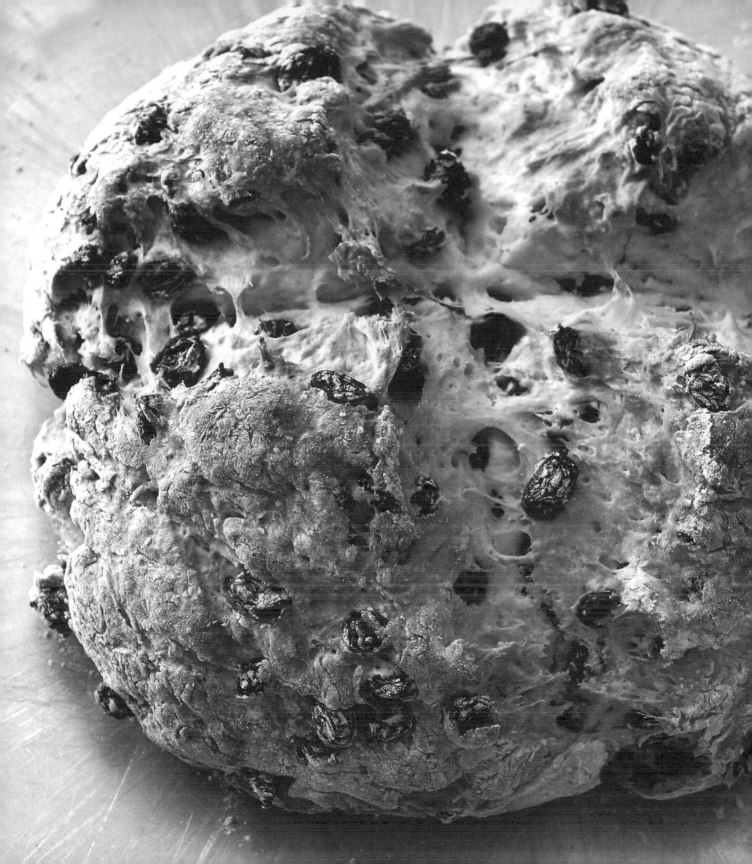

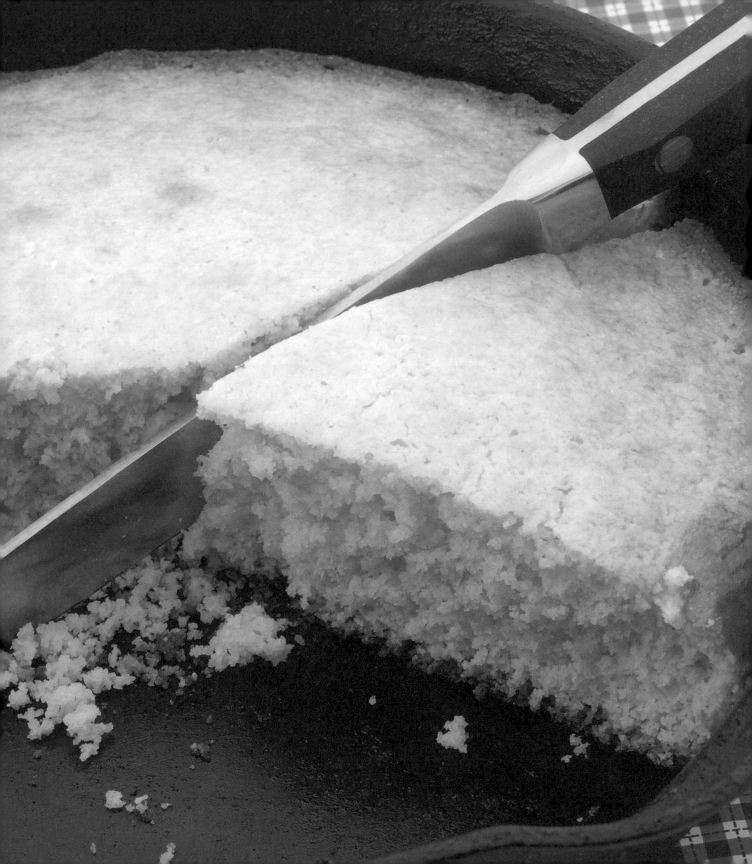

Cornbread

If you have a well-seasoned cast iron skillet around, you can bake the cornbread right in it and bring it to the table. This is an all-purpose recipe that really goes with any entree and is as at home on the breakfast table as on the dinner table.

Yield: 6–8 servings

Active time: 10 minutes

Start to finish: 30 minutes

1 cup fine yellow gluten-free cornmeal

⅔ cup white rice flour

¼ cup potato starch

2 tablespoons tapioca flour

2 tablespoons granulated sugar

1½ teaspoons gluten-free baking powder

1 teaspoon xanthan gum

½ teaspoon baking soda

¼ teaspoon salt

2 large eggs

¾ cups buttermilk, well shaken

½ cup creamed corn

5 tablespoons unsalted butter, melted

1. Preheat the oven to 425°F, and grease a 9x9-inch baking pan generously.

2. Whisk together cornmeal, rice flour, potato starch, tapioca flour, sugar, baking powder, xanthan gum, baking soda, and salt in a large mixing bowl. Whisk together eggs, buttermilk, creamed corn, and butter in a small bowl. Add buttermilk mixture to cornmeal mixture, and stir batter until just blended.

3. Heat the greased pan in the oven for 3 minutes, or until it is very hot. Remove the pan from the oven, and spread batter in it evenly. Bake cornbread in the middle of the oven for 15 minutes, or until top is pale golden and the sides begin to pull away from the edges of the pan.

4. Allow cornbread to cool for 5 minutes, then turn it out onto a rack. Cut into pieces, and serve hot or at room temperature.

Note: Cornbread is best eaten within a few hours of baking.

Variations:
* *Add 1 cup dried cranberries and 1½ tablespoons crushed fennel seeds to the batter.*
* *Add 1 cup fresh or frozen raspberries to the batter. If using frozen raspberries do not thaw them before using.*
* *Add ½ cup crumbled cooked bacon, and substitute bacon grease for the melted butter.*
* *Add ½ cup finely chopped pimiento to the batter.*
* *Add ½ cup chopped dried apricots and ½ teaspoon Chinese five-spice powder to the batter.*
* *Add ½ cup toasted chopped pecans and ½ teaspoon ground cinnamon to the batter and substitute firmly packed dark brown sugar for the granulated sugar.*

If you don't use buttermilk very often, it's a waste of money to buy a quart to use less than half in a recipe. Instead, buy buttermilk powder. It's shelved with the baking ingredients in the supermarket. Refrigerate it once opened.

Gooey Pecan Sticky Buns

I'm now making sticky buns for the third generation of my family, and it wouldn't be a holiday without them. These are the epitome of a festive breakfast.

Yield: 24 buns

Active time: 30 minutes

Start to finish: 3½ hours

Dough:

1 cup brown rice flour

1 cup tapioca flour

3¾ cups cornstarch

2 tablespoons xanthan gum

2 (¼-ounce) packages active dry yeast

1 teaspoon salt

2 cups warm whole milk (110–115°F)

1 cup honey

4 large eggs, at room temperature

1 cup (2 sticks) unsalted butter, melted and cooled

2 teaspoons pure vanilla extract

Glaze and Filling:

4 cups chopped pecans, divided

¾ cup (1½ sticks) unsalted butter, melted, divided

2½ cups firmly packed light brown sugar, divided

½ cup light corn syrup

3 tablespoons heavy cream

3 teaspoons ground cinnamon

½ teaspoon freshly grated nutmeg

½ teaspoon ground ginger

Vegetable oil spray

1. Combine brown rice flour, tapioca flour, cornstarch, xanthan gum, yeast, and salt in a mixing bowl. Whisk well.

2. Combine milk, honey, eggs, butter, and vanilla in the mixing bowl of a standard mixer fitted with the paddle attachment. Beat at medium speed for 1 minute. Reduce the speed to low, and add flour mixture. Beat at low speed for 2 minutes.

3. Cover the bowl loosely with a sheet of plastic wrap, and place it in a warm spot for 1–2 hours, or until dough is doubled in bulk.

4. While dough rises, make glaze and filling. Preheat the oven to 350°F. Toast pecans on a baking sheet for 5–7 minutes, or until browned.

5. Combine 9 tablespoons butter, 1½ cups sugar, corn syrup, and cream in a small saucepan. Bring to a boil over medium heat, stirring occasionally. Grease 3 (9-inch) round cake pans with vegetable oil spray. Divide glaze into the bottoms of the pans, and tilt to spread glaze evenly. Sprinkle 1 cup of chopped pecans over glaze in each pan.

6. For filling, combine remaining pecans, remaining butter, remaining sugar, cinnamon, nutmeg, and ginger in a mixing bowl.

7. Spray your hands with vegetable oil spray. Divide dough into 3 parts. Sprinkle a counter and rolling pin heavily with brown rice flour. Roll dough into a rectangle approximately 10x15 inches; this is the size of an average cookie sheet. Sprinkle rectangle with ⅓ of the filling, and roll it beginning with the long side. Cut log into 8 pieces, and space them evenly on top of the glaze. Flatten them lightly until they barely touch each other. Repeat with the remaining dough portions and filling.

8. Cover pans lightly with a tea towel, and allow them to rise for 1 hour, or until very puffy.

9. While buns rise, preheat the oven to 350°F. Bake buns for 30–35 minutes, or until brown. Remove the pans from the oven, and invert buns onto a platter. Scrape any glaze remaining in the pan on top of the buns, and serve warm.

Note: While best right out of the oven, the buns can be baked up to 2 days in advance and kept at room temperature, tightly covered. Reheat them, covered with foil, in a 300°F oven for 8–10 minutes.

Variation:
* *Substitute maple sugar for the light brown sugar, and substitute walnuts for the pecans.*

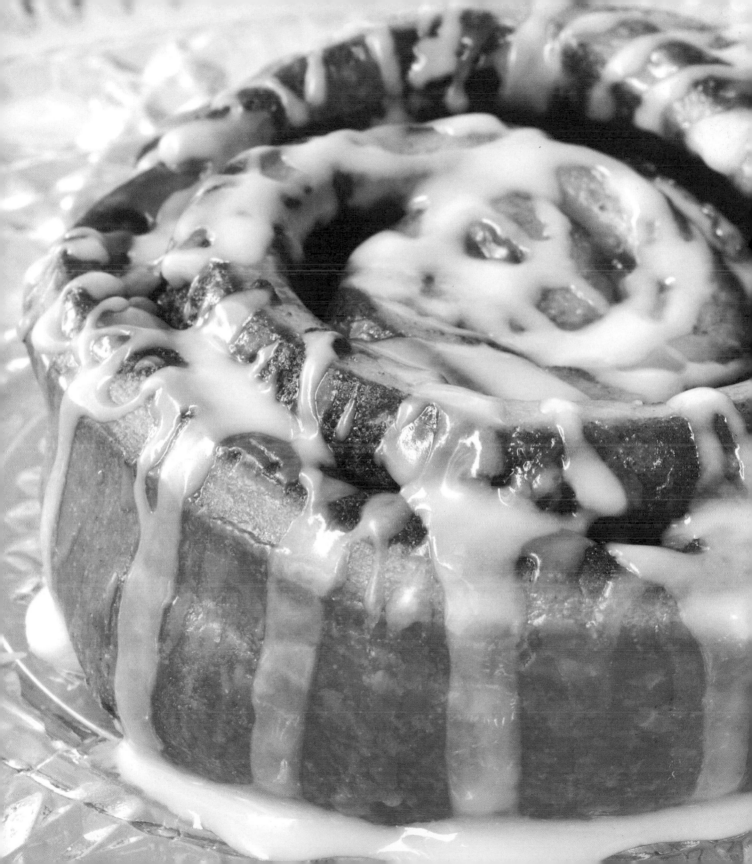

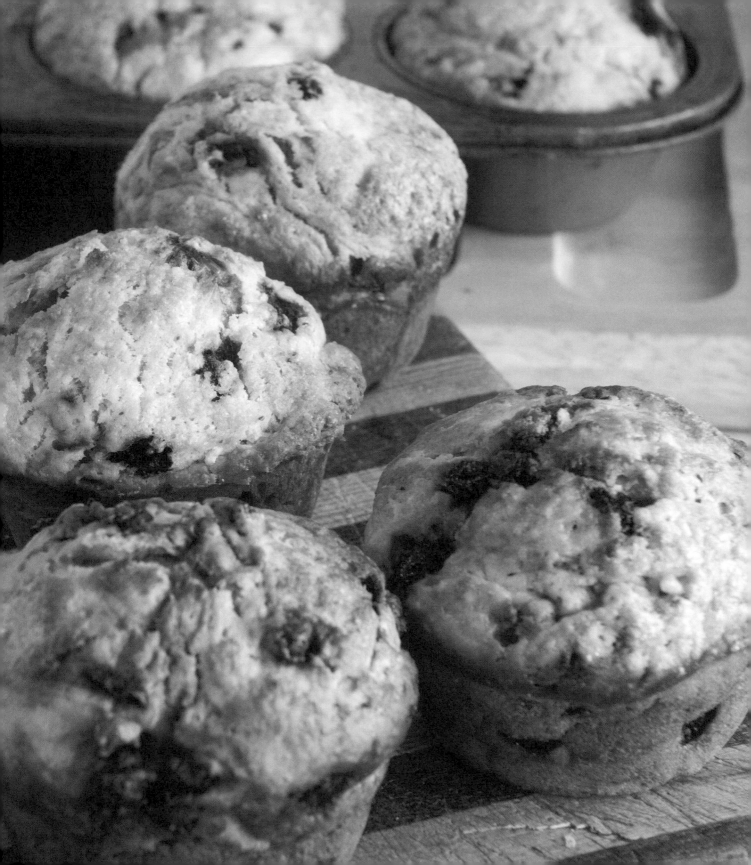

Blueberry Muffins

The combination of chopped and whole berries in these vivid purple muffins delivers the maximum blueberry flavor, and they can easily be made with frozen berries off-season.

Yield: 12 muffins

Active time: 10 minutes

Start to finish: 30 minutes

2 cups fresh blueberries

1 cup brown rice flour

⅔ cup potato starch

¼ cup tapioca flour

1 tablespoon gluten-free baking powder

½ cup granulated sugar

½ teaspoon ground cinnamon

½ teaspoon salt

½ teaspoon baking soda

½ teaspoon xanthan gum

1 cup buttermilk, shaken well

1 large egg, lightly beaten

6 tablespoons unsalted butter, melted

½ teaspoon pure vanilla extract

1. Preheat the oven to 400°F, and grease a 12-cup muffin pan; you can also use paper liners and spray the top of the pan with vegetable oil spray. Place 1 cup blueberries in a food processor fitted with the steel blade, and chop finely using on-and-off pulsing. Set aside.

2. Combine rice flour, potato starch, tapioca flour, baking powder, sugar, cinnamon, salt, baking soda, and xanthan gum in a large mixing bowl, and whisk well. Add chopped berries, buttermilk, egg, butter, and vanilla. Stir gently to wet flour, but do not whisk until smooth; batter should be lumpy. Fold in remaining blueberries. Fill each prepared cup ⅔ full.

3. Bake muffins for 18–20 minutes, or until a toothpick inserted in the center comes out clean. Place muffin pan on a cooling rack for 10 minutes, then serve—either hot or at room temperature.

Variations:
* *Substitute raspberries or blackberries for the blueberries.*
* *Add the grated zest and juice of 1 lemon to the batter, and omit the vanilla.*

> Frozen fruit can be used in baking, but always use it in its frozen state. If you allow it to thaw, it will not measure correctly, and it will create too much liquid in a recipe.

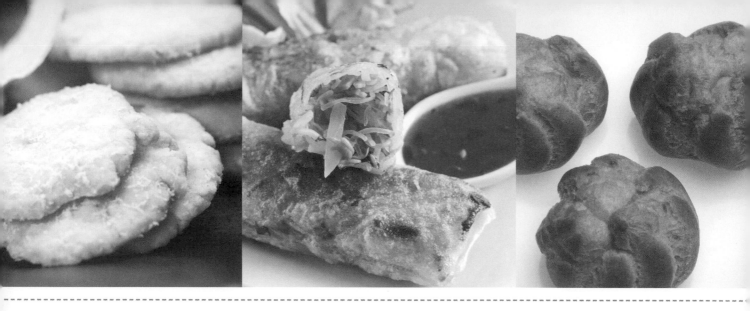

CHAPTER 5:

Savory Nibbles for Holiday Entertaining

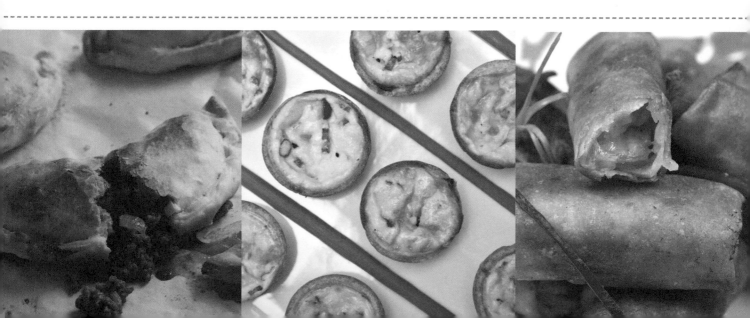

It's not just the dessert table and breadbasket that present potential problems for those following a gluten-free diet. There are all those canapés and other hors d'oeuvres passed at parties too. Anything that sits on top of a round of toast, or a slice of bread, or is encased in pastry most likely contains gluten, which is why those who must avoid it are the ones hanging around the crudité basket or eating cheese wedges with their fingers.

But that not need be the case. In this chapter you'll find fantastic crispy and crunchy hors d'oeuvres that everyone at the party will love. These recipes are drawn from many cuisines— from subtly seasoned classic French to lusty Latin and Asian options. Although I do believe that a dinner menu should not mix parts of the world, I think that the sky is the limit when it comes to hors d'oeuvres.

This chapter includes basic recipes for gluten-free versions of empanada dough and tartlet dough. These will make it possible for you to modify some of your favorite hors d'oeuvre recipes—including quiches and any turnovers—to make them gluten-free.

Readymade Wrappers

A stalwart for gluten-free hors d'oeuvres are the rice paper pancakes used in Thai and Vietnamese cooking. They can be substituted in savory and sweet dishes for crispy sheets of phyllo dough, which at present does not have a commercial gluten-free version and is almost impossible to make. The thin pancakes must be quickly soaked in water to make them pliable enough to roll around a filling, but then they crisp beautifully when baked in a hot oven. You'll find recipes using them in this chapter, and also in Chapter 3 for individual sweet pastries. It takes a few minutes to become proficient at handling the rice paper pancakes, but once you've mastered the skill you'll find how easy they are to use, and how versatile too.

Even people not following a gluten-free diet are always appreciative of vegetables as wrappers as a diet aide during the calorie-filled holidays too. For anything from cheeses to dips, put out a plate of Belgian endive leaves or small cups of Bibb lettuce as alternatives to crackers or bread.

Frico (Parmesan Crisps)

These are always a hit with guests, and there are so many ways to serve them. Pass them as a nibble with cocktails, or serve them on the rim of a salad plate.

Yield: 36 crisps

Active time: 10 minutes

Start to finish: 25 minutes

2 cups freshly grated
Parmesan cheese

2 tablespoons
brown rice flour

2 teaspoons cornstarch

Pinch cayenne

1. Preheat the oven to 375°F. Line two baking sheets with parchment paper or silicone baking mats.

2. Combine cheese, rice flour, cornstarch, and cayenne in a mixing bowl. Place 1-tablespoon portions on the baking sheets, leaving 1½ inches between mounds, tossing the cheese mixture frequently to keep the flour evenly distributed. Press mounds flat with your fingers or the back of a spatula.

3. Bake for 9–12 minutes, or until brown. Cool crisps on the baking sheets for 2 minutes, then remove them with a slotted spatula to a cooling rack to cool completely.

Note: The crisps keep at room temperature for up to a week in an airtight container.

Variations:
* *Substitute herbes de Provence or Italian seasoning for the cayenne.*
* *Substitute Peccorino Romano or goat Cheddar for the Parmesan.*

> The reason why authentic Parmesan and satiny prosciutto go so well together is that the pigs eat the whey created when making the cheese. True Parmesan can only be produced in a small part of one region of Italy.

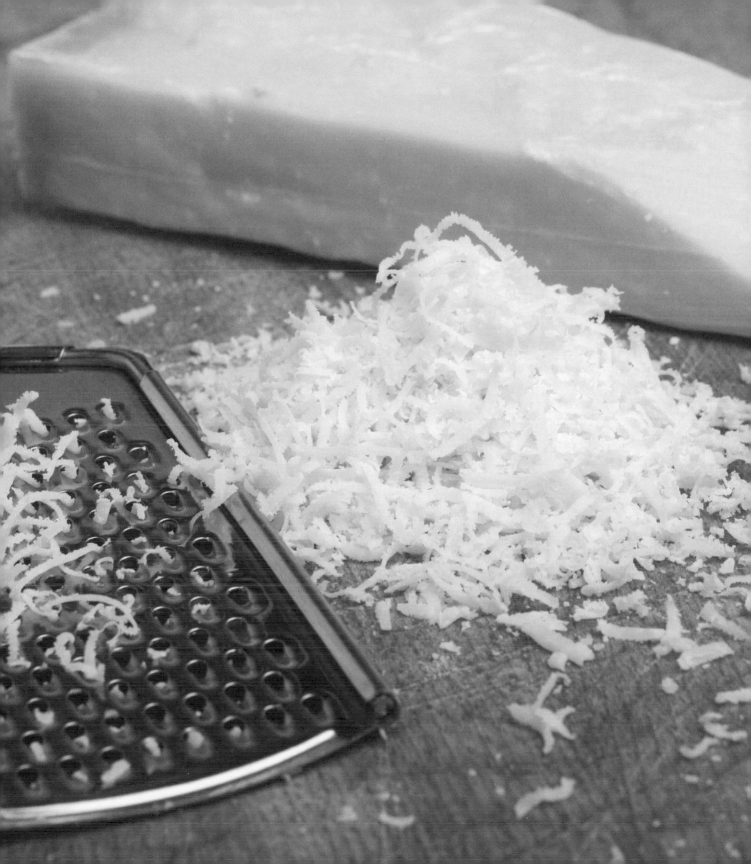

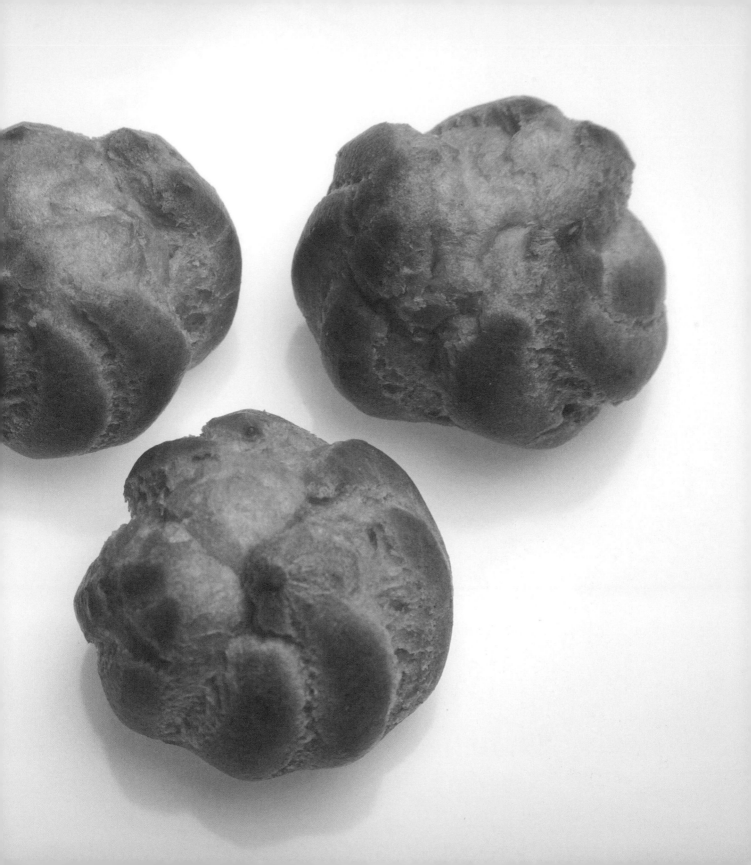

Gougères

These cheese puffs hail from the Burgundy region of France, and they're crispy and ethereally light.

Yield: 40 puffs

Active time: 20 minutes

Start to finish: 45 minutes

½ cup brown rice flour

¼ cup potato starch

¼ cup tapioca flour

¼ teaspoon xanthan gum

1 cup chicken stock

6 tablespoons (¾ stick) unsalted butter, cut into thin slices

½ teaspoon salt

¼ teaspoon freshly grated nutmeg

Pinch of freshly grated white pepper

4 large eggs, at room temperature

1¼ cups grated Gruyère cheese, divided

1. Preheat the oven to 400° F, and line two baking sheets with parchment paper or silicone baking mats.

2. Combine rice flour, potato starch, tapioca flour, and xanthan gum in a mixing bowl. Whisk well.

3. Combine stock, butter, salt, nutmeg, and pepper in a small saucepan, and bring to a boil over medium-high heat, stirring occasionally. Remove the pan from the heat, and add rice flour mixture all at once. Using a wooden paddle or wide wooden spoon, beat dry ingredients into liquid until smooth. Then place the saucepan over high heat and beat mixture constantly for 1–2 minutes, or until it forms a mass that leaves the sides of the pan and begins to film the bottom of the pot.

4. Transfer mixture to a food processor fitted with the steel blade. Add eggs, 1 at a time, beating well between each addition and scraping the sides of the work bowl between each addition. Then add 1 cup cheese, and mix well again.

5. Using a soupspoon dipped in cold water, form dough into mounds 1 inch in diameter and 1 inch high on the baking sheets, allowing 2 inches between puffs. Sprinkle remaining cheese on top of puffs.

6. Bake puffs for 18–20 minutes, or until puffs are golden brown and crusty to the touch. Remove the pans from the oven, and using the tip of a paring knife, cut a slit in the side of the puff to allow the steam to escape. Turn off the oven, and place baked puffs back into the oven with the oven door ajar for 5 minutes to finish crisping. Remove puffs from the oven, and serve immediately.

Note: The puffs can be made up to 2 days in advance and refrigerated, tightly covered; they can also be frozen for up to 2 weeks. Reheat chilled puffs in a 350°F oven for 5–7 minutes and frozen puffs for 12–15 minutes.

Variations:
* *Substitute sharp Cheddar, Swiss cheese, or Manchego for the Gruyère.*
* *Add ¼ cup finely chopped cooked bacon or ham to the dough.*
* *Add 2 tablespoons chopped fresh basil and 2 tablespoons finely chopped sun-dried tomatoes to the dough.*

Cheddar Wafers

Admittedly, including crushed potato chips in an ingredient list is unusual, but they make these the crunchiest as well as most flavorful cheese crackers you'll ever taste.

Yield: 2 dozen

Active time: 15 minutes

Start to finish: 35 minutes

1 (5.5-ounce) bag
potato chips

1½ cups grated sharp
Cheddar cheese

5 tablespoons unsalted
butter, melted

¼ cup brown rice flour

2 tablespoons potato starch

½ teaspoon cayenne,
or to taste

1. Preheat the oven to 350°F. Line two baking sheets with parchment paper or silicone baking mats.

2. Chop potato chips coarsely in a food processor fitted with the steel blade, using on-and-off pulsing. Scrape crumbs into a bowl and add cheese, butter, flour, potato starch, and cayenne. Stir until mixture is combined and holds together when pressed in the palm of your hand.

3. Form 1 tablespoon portions of mixture into a ball. Place it on baking sheets and flatten it into a circle with the bottom of a glass dipped in rice flour or with your fingers. Repeat with remaining dough, leaving 1 inch between the circles.

4. Bake for 15–18 minutes, or until browned. Cool crackers on the baking sheet for 2 minutes, then transfer them to a cooling rack with a spatula to cool completely. Serve at room temperature.

Note: The crackers can be made 2 days in advance and kept at room temperature in an airtight container.

Variations:
* *Substitute your favorite flavor of potato chips—such as sour cream and onion or barbecue—for the plain chips, and omit the cayenne.*
* *Substitute Gruyère, Monterey Jack, or Jalapeño Jack for the cheddar.*

> **Cheddar is named for the village in Somerset, in the southwestern corner of England. It's rumored that the Romans may have brought the recipe from the Cantal region of France, where a similar cheese is produced. Cheddar has ben made in England since the twelfth century, and traditional Cheddar is made within thirty miles of Wells Cathedral and aged in caves in an area on the outskirts of the village called Cheddar Gorge.**

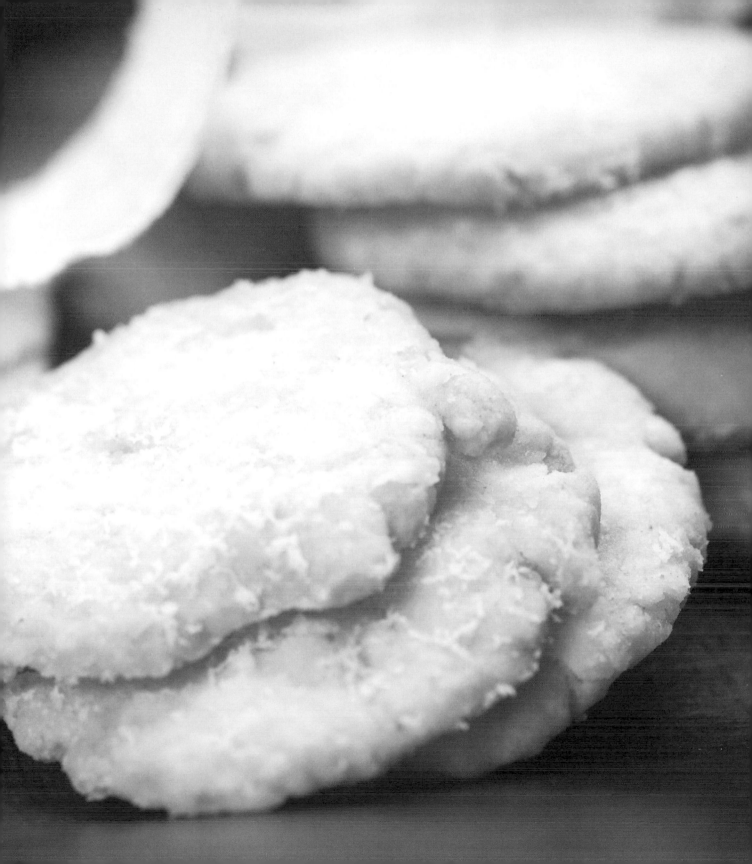

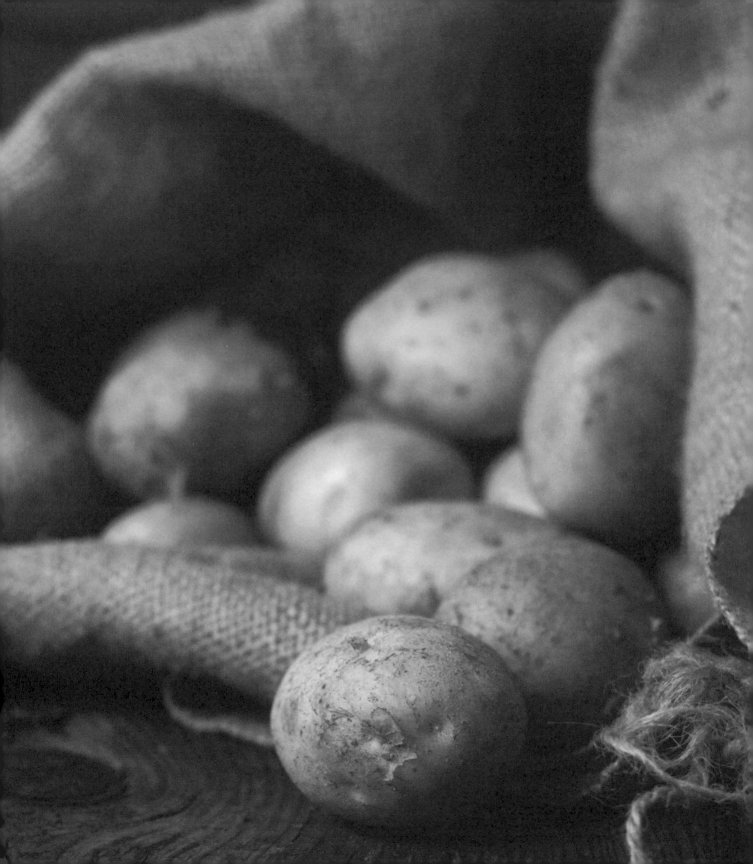

Potato and Cheese Sticks

These tasty and crunchy morsels are another classic French treat, and they're much easier to make than traditional cheese sticks. And they can be done in advance, which is great for party planning.

Yield: 3 dozen

Active time: 15 minutes

Start to finish: 40 minutes

½ pound russet potatoes, peeled and cut into 1-inch dice

½ cup brown rice flour

¼ cup potato starch

2 tablespoons tapioca flour

⅛ teaspoon xanthan gum

¼ pound (1 stick) unsalted butter, softened and cut into small pieces

1 large egg, lightly beaten

1 cup grated sharp cheddar cheese

Salt and freshly ground black pepper to taste

Cayenne to taste

1. Preheat the oven to 425°F, line two baking sheets with heavy-duty aluminum foil, and grease the foil.

2. Boil potatoes in salted water for 10–12 minutes, or until very tender when pierced with a knife. Drain potatoes, shaking the colander vigorously to extract as much liquid as possible. Return potatoes to the pan, and mash well or put potatoes through a ricer. Cook mashed potatoes over low heat for 1–2 minutes, or until they begin to form a film on the bottom of the pan.

3. Combine rice flour, potato starch, tapioca flour, and xanthan gum in a bowl. Whisk well. Beat dry mixture, then add butter, bit by bit, beating well to ensure that butter melts; place the pan over low heat if butter is not melting in. Beat in egg and cheese, and season to taste with salt, pepper, and cayenne.

4. Transfer potato mixture to a pastry bag fitted with a ½-inch fluted tip, and pipe out dough into 2-inch lengths. Bake sticks for 12–15 minutes, or until browned. Serve hot.

Note: The sticks can be prepared up to 2 days in advance and refrigerated, tightly covered. Reheat them in a 375°F oven for 3–5 minutes, or until hot. Undercook sticks slightly if you're planning on reheating them.

Variations:
* *Substitute Swiss cheese for the cheddar cheese.*
* *Add 1 teaspoon Italian seasoning or herbes de Provence to the potato mixture.*

The best place to store eggs is in their cardboard carton. The carton helps prevent moisture loss, and it shields the eggs from absorbing odors from other foods. If you're not sure if your eggs are fresh, submerge them in a bowl of cool water. If they stay on the bottom, they're fine. If they float to the top, it shows they're old because eggs develop an air pocket at one end as they age.

Sauerkraut Balls with Mustard Sauce

Sauerkraut itself is German, but these Sauerkraut Balls are a treasured treat of Midwestern cooking due to the large number of German settlers in the region. The sauerkraut is mixed with potato, and the dipping sauce has lots of mustard.

Yield: 4 dozen

Active time: 20 minutes

Start to finish: 30 minutes

1 pound potatoes, peeled

1 pound sauerkraut, drained well

2 large eggs

¾ cup whole grain Dijon mustard, divided

3 scallions, white parts and 2 inches of green tops, rinsed, trimmed, and chopped

2 tablespoons chopped fresh parsley

Salt and freshly ground black pepper to taste

1 cup plain gluten-free breadcrumbs

½ cup mayonnaise

½ cup sour cream

Vegetable oil spray

1. Preheat the oven to 425°F. Cover two baking sheets with heavy-duty aluminum foil, and coat the foil with vegetable oil spray.

2. Dice potatoes into 1-inch cubes, and boil in salted water for 10–15 minutes, or until very tender. Drain potatoes, shaking them in a colander to get out as much water as possible. Mash potatoes until smooth, and set aside.

3. While potatoes boil, soak sauerkraut in cold water, changing the water every 3 minutes for a total of 3 times. Drain sauerkraut, pressing with the back of a spoon to extract as much liquid as possible, and coarsely chop sauerkraut.

4. Whisk eggs and ¼ cup mustard in a mixing bowl, and add potatoes, sauerkraut, scallions, and parsley. Mix well, and season to taste with salt and pepper.

5. Place breadcrumbs in a shallow bowl. Form sauerkraut mixture into 1-inch balls, roll balls in breadcrumbs, and arrange balls on the prepared baking sheets. Spray balls heavily with vegetable oil spray. Bake balls for 5–7 minutes, or until crispy.

6. While balls bake, mix remaining ½ cup mustard with mayonnaise and sour cream, and whisk well. Serve balls hot, with sauce on the side.

Note: The sauerkraut balls can be prepared for baking up to 1 day in advance and refrigerated, tightly covered. Add 2 minutes to the baking time if chilled.

Variations:
* *Add ½ cup finely chopped ham or cooked sausage, such as smoked kielbasa.*
* *Add ½ cup grated cheese, such as cheddar or smoked cheddar.*

> You've probably noticed that I use a lot of aluminum foil, and, no, I don't own stock in any company that makes it. Lining any pan destined for the oven with aluminum foil cuts cleanup time significantly. The only times not to use it are when you are working on top of the stove or when you plan to use the drippings in an oven pan to make gravy.

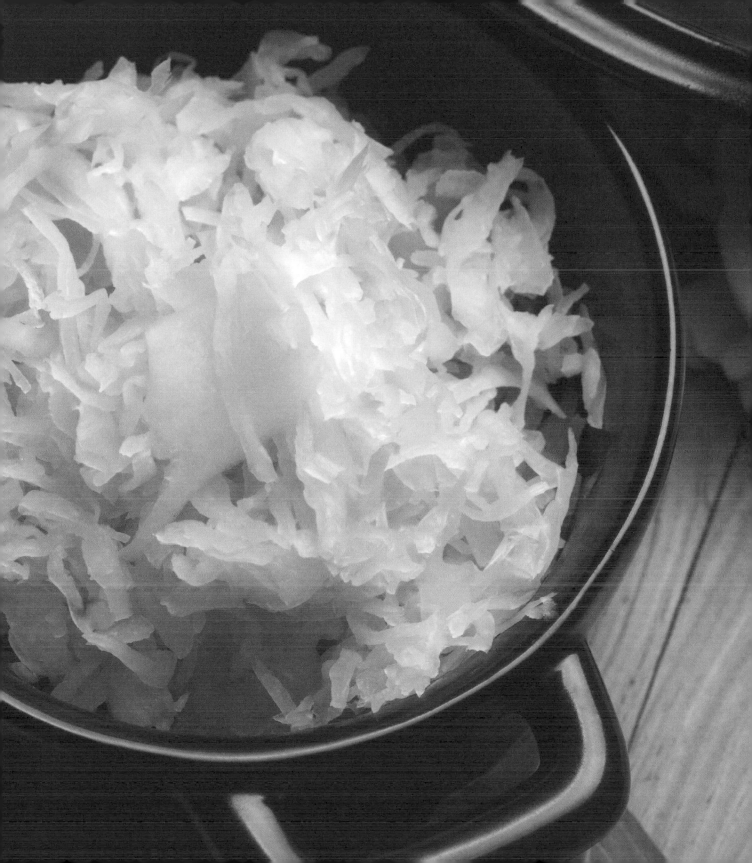

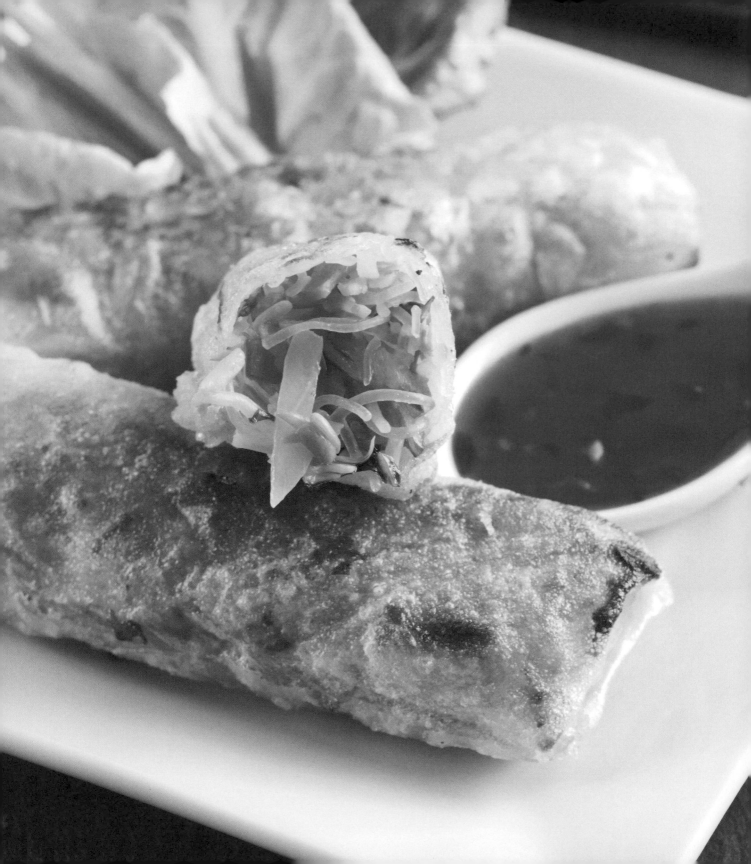

Vietnamese Spring Rolls

Cha Gio, *crispy Vietnamese spring rolls made with dried shiitake mushrooms, bean sprouts, and pork, are one of my favorite dishes, and by baking instead of frying them they are much lighter and quicker to prepare.*

Yield: 18 rolls

Active time: 35 minutes

Start to finish: 55 minutes

5 large dried shiitake mushrooms

1 ounce bean thread noodles

½ pound ground pork

1 cup fresh bean sprouts, rinsed and cut into 1-inch lengths

½ cup shredded carrot

½ cup chopped scallions, white part and 4 inches of green tops

4 garlic cloves, minced

3 tablespoons fish sauce

2 large eggs, lightly beaten

½ cup granulated sugar, divided

Salt and freshly ground black pepper to taste

18 (8-inch) rice paper pancakes

Vegetable oil spray

1. Soak dried mushrooms and bean thread noodles in separate bowls of very hot tap water for 30 minutes. Remove mushrooms, and squeeze well to extract as much water as possible. Discard stems, and finely chop mushrooms. Drain bean thread noodles. Place them on a cutting board in a long log shape, and cut into 1-inch pieces. Measure out ½ cup, and discard any additional.

2. Preheat the oven to 400°F. Cover a baking sheet with heavy-duty aluminum foil, and spray the foil with vegetable oil spray.

3. Place mushrooms and noodles in a mixing bowl, and add pork, bean sprouts, carrot, scallions, garlic, fish sauce, eggs, and 1 teaspoon sugar. Mix well, and season to taste with salt and pepper.

4. Fill a wide mixing bowl with very hot tap water, and stir in remaining sugar until dissolved. Place a damp tea towel in front of you on the counter. Place rice paper pancakes on a plate, and cover with a barely damp towel.

5. Fill 1 rice paper pancake at a time, keeping remainder covered. Totally immerse pancake in the hot water for 2 seconds. Remove it and place it on the damp tea towel; it will become pliable within a few seconds. Gently fold front edge of pancake one-third of the way to the top. Place about 2 tablespoons of filling on the folded up portion, and shape it into a log, leaving a 2-inch margin on each side. Lightly spray unfilled pancake with vegetable oil spray. Fold sides over filling, and roll tightly but gently, beginning with the filled side. Place roll on the baking sheet, and continue to fill remaining pancakes in the same manner.

6. Spray tops and sides of rolls with vegetable oil spray, and place them in the center of the preheated oven. Bake for 12 minutes, then turn rolls gently with tongs, and bake another 10–12 minutes, or until rolls are browned. Remove the pan from the oven, and blot rolls with paper towels. Slice each in half on the diagonal, and serve immediately.

Note: The filling can be prepared up to 1 day in advance and refrigerated, tightly covered. The rolls can be baked up to 2 days in advance. Reheat them in a 350°F oven for 5–7 minutes, or until hot and crisp.

Variation:
* *Substitute ground turkey or ground chicken for the pork.*

Spicy Shrimp and Cabbage Spring Rolls

These are a light and luscious hors d'oeuvre. The combination of seasonings enliven the crispy cabbage. You'll find yourself serving them on many occasions when the meal is not Asian too.

Yield: 18 rolls

Active time: 25 minutes

Start to finish: 55 minutes

2 tablespoons Asian
sesame oil

1 tablespoon grated
fresh ginger

3 garlic cloves, minced

1 jalapeño or serrano chile,
seeds and ribs removed,
and chopped

1 carrot, cut into fine julienne

6 scallions, white parts and 4
inches of green tops, chopped

2 cups firmly packed
shredded bok choy or
Napa cabbage

¼ cup chopped fresh cilantro

¾ pound cooked shrimp,
chopped

2 tablespoons Chinese
rice wine or dry Sherry

1 tablespoon reduced-sodium
soy sauce

Salt and freshly ground black
pepper to taste

½ cup granulated sugar

18 (8-inch) rice paper
pancakes

Vegetable oil spray

1. Preheat the oven to 400°F. Cover a baking sheet with heavy-duty aluminum foil, and spray the foil with vegetable oil spray.

2. Heat sesame oil in a wok or large skillet over high heat. Add ginger, garlic, and chile. Cook, stirring constantly, for 1 minute. Add carrot, scallions, and cabbage. Cook for 1½–2 minutes, or until cabbage wilts. Stir in cilantro, shrimp, wine, and soy sauce. Remove the pan from the heat. Season to taste with salt and pepper.

3. Fill a wide mixing bowl with very hot tap water, and stir in remaining sugar until dissolved. Place a damp tea towel in front of you on the counter. Place rice paper pancakes on a plate, and cover with a barely damp towel.

4. Fill 1 rice paper pancake at a time, keeping remainder covered. Totally immerse pancake in the hot water for 2 seconds. Remove it and place it on the damp tea towel; it will become pliable within a few seconds. Gently fold front edge of pancake one-third of the way to the top. Place about 2 tablespoons of filling on the folded up portion, and shape it into a log, leaving a 2-inch margin on each side. Lightly spray unfilled pancake with vegetable oil spray. Fold sides over filling, and roll tightly but gently, beginning with the filled side. Place roll on the baking sheet, and continue to fill remaining pancakes in the same manner.

5. Spray tops and sides of rolls with vegetable oil spray, and place them in the center of the preheated oven. Bake for 12 minutes, then turn rolls gently with tongs, and bake an additional 10–12 minutes, or until rolls are browned. Remove the pan from the oven, and blot rolls with paper towels. Slice each in half on the diagonal, and serve immediately.

Note: The filling can be prepared up to 1 day in advance and refrigerated, tightly covered. The rolls can be baked up to 2 days in advance. Reheat them in a 350°F oven for 5–7 minutes, or until hot and crisp.

Variations:
* *Substitute lump crabmeat or lobster for the shrimp.*
* *Substitute shredded broccoli for the cabbage.*

> **It's common to see jalapeño and serrano chilies given as recipe options in the same quantity although serrano peppers are much smaller. They are also much hotter, so the larger jalapeño and the small serrano produce the same amount of heat.**

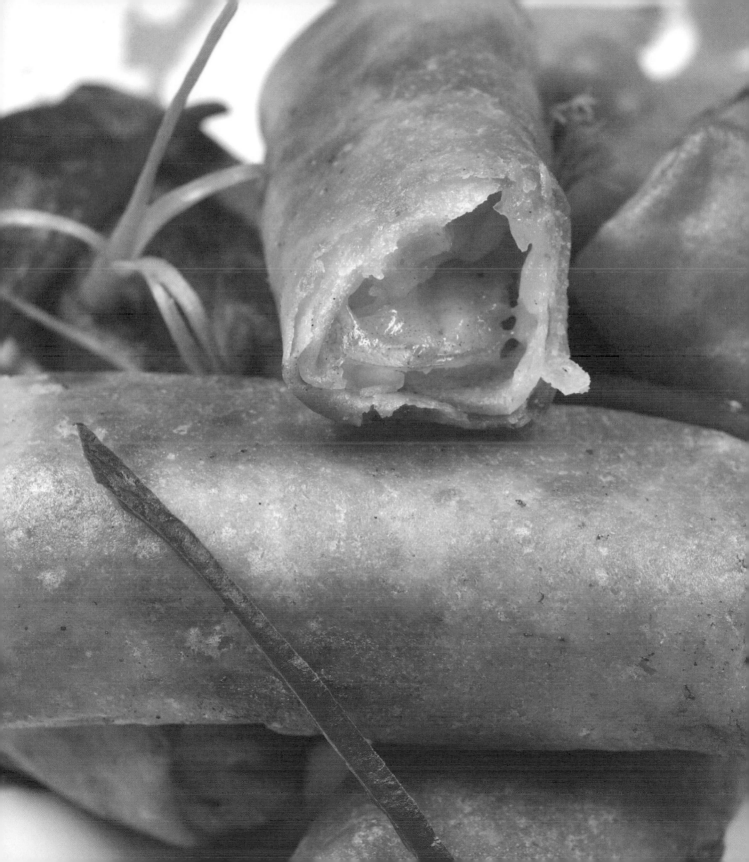

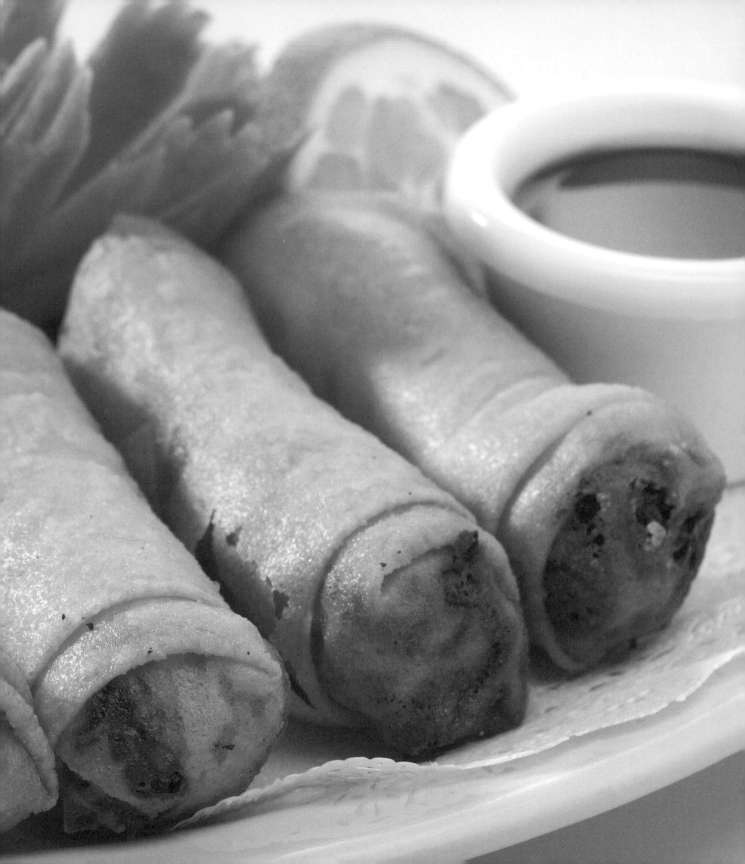

Truffled Wild Mushroom Rolls

These crunchy rolls are a great example of Asian Fusion cooking. While the wrappers and method are Asian, the mélange of woodsy wild mushrooms are drawn from Western cuisines. The final brushing with aromatic truffle oil elevates them even higher.

Yield: 18 rolls

Active time: 25 minutes

Start to finish: 55 minutes

½ cup dried porcini mushrooms

½ cup boiling water

3 tablespoons unsalted butter

2 shallots, chopped

2 garlic cloves, minced

½ pound assorted fresh wild mushrooms (such as shiitake, Portobello, and cremini), finely chopped

¼ cup dry sherry

2 tablespoons chopped fresh parsley

2 teaspoons fresh thyme or ½ teaspoon dried

Salt and freshly ground black pepper to taste

18 (8-inch) rice paper pancakes

½ cup granulated sugar

Vegetable oil spray

2 tablespoons truffle oil

1. Combine dried mushrooms and boiling water, pushing them down into the water. Soak for 10 minutes, then drain mushrooms, reserving soaking liquid, and chop mushrooms. Strain soaking liquid through a sieve lined with a paper coffee filter or a paper towel. Set aside.

2. Heat butter in a large skillet over medium-high heat. Add shallots and garlic, and cook, stirring frequently, for 3 minutes, or until shallots are translucent. Add chopped mushrooms, and cook for 2 minutes. Add rehydrated mushrooms, soaking liquid, sherry, parsley, and thyme. Cook over high heat, stirring occasionally, for 5–7 minutes, or until liquid evaporates. Season to taste with salt and pepper. Spread onto a plate, and chill for 10 minutes, or until cold.

3. Preheat the oven to 400°F. Cover a baking sheet with heavy-duty aluminum foil, and spray the foil with vegetable oil spray.

4. Fill a wide mixing bowl with very hot tap water, and stir in sugar until dissolved. Place a damp tea towel in front of you on the counter. Place rice paper pancakes on a plate, and cover with a barely damp towel.

5. Fill 1 rice paper pancake at a time, keeping remainder covered. Totally immerse pancake in the hot water for 2 seconds. Remove it and place it on the damp tea towel; it will become pliable within a few seconds. Gently fold front edge of pancake one-third of the way to the top. Place about 2 tablespoons of filling on the folded up portion, and shape it into a log, leaving a 2-inch margin on each side. Lightly spray unfilled pancake with vegetable oil spray. Fold sides over filling, and roll tightly but gently, beginning with the filled side. Place roll on the baking sheet, and continue to fill remaining pancakes in the same manner.

6. Spray tops and sides of rolls with vegetable oil spray, and place them in the center of the preheated oven. Bake for 12 minutes, then turn rolls gently with tongs, and bake an additional 10–12 minutes, or until rolls are browned. Remove the pan from the oven, and blot rolls with paper towels. Brush each roll with truffle oil. Slice each in half on the diagonal, and serve immediately.

Note: The filling can be prepared up to 1 day in advance and refrigerated, tightly covered. The rolls can be baked up to 2 days in advance. Reheat them in a 350°F oven for 5–7 minutes, or until hot and crisp.

Variation:
❋ *Add 3 tablespoons freshly grated Parmesan cheese or crumbled feta to the filling.*

129

Empanada Dough

This is a gluten-free version of an authentic Mexican dough. It contains a specific form of cornmeal, and the pastry tastes similar to the wrappers for tamales.

Yield: enough for 2 dozen empanadas

Active time: 15 minutes

Start to finish: 45 minutes

1 cup brown rice flour

¼ cup potato starch

¼ cup tapioca flour

1 cup gluten-free masa harina

1 teaspoon gluten-free baking powder

½ teaspoon xanthan gum

½ teaspoon salt

½ cup (1 stick) unsalted butter, melted and cooled

1. Combine brown rice flour, potato starch, tapioca flour, masa harina, baking powder, and xanthan gum in a large bowl. Whisk well.

2. Stir in butter. Gradually add ½ to ¾ cup water, working it into dough with your hands. Dough should be easy to handle and not sticky. Add more masa harina if dough is sticky. Divide dough in half, and form into a flat "pancake." Wrap each "pancake" in plastic wrap, and chill for at least 30 minutes. Roll and fill dough per instructions in individual recipes.

Note: The dough can be refrigerated for up to 1 day.

Variation:
✳ *Add ½ to 1 teaspoon cayenne to mixture for a spicy pastry dough.*

> To make masa harina, field corn is dried and then treated in a solution of lime and water called slaked lime. This loosens the hulls from the kernels and softens the corn. In addition, the lime reacts with the corn so that the nutrient niacin can be assimilated by the digestive tract. The soaked maize is then washed, and the wet corn is ground into dough, called masa. It is this fresh masa, when dried and powdered, which becomes masa harina.

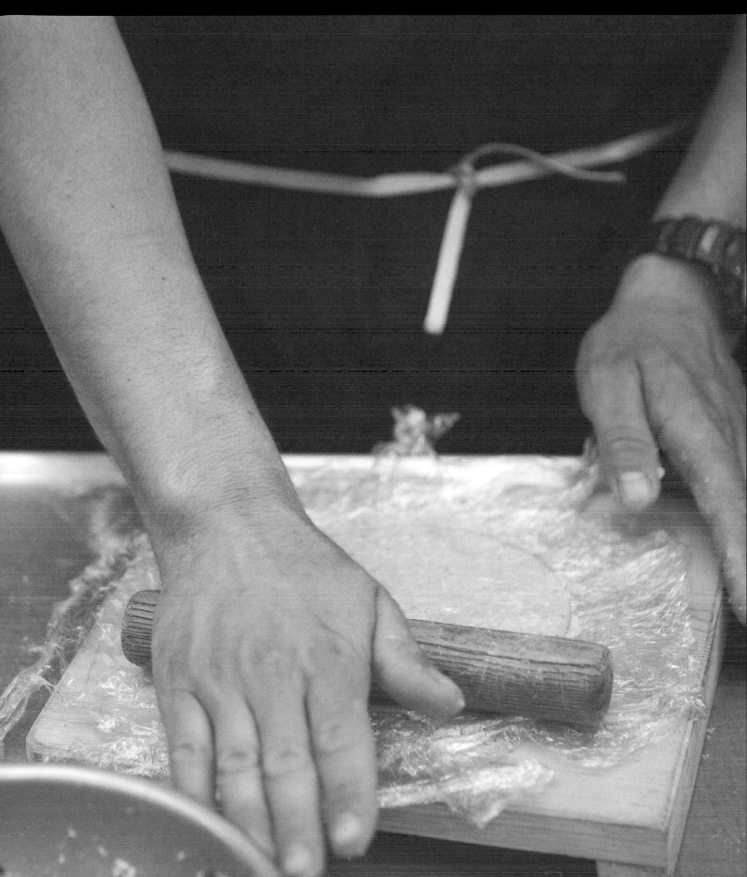

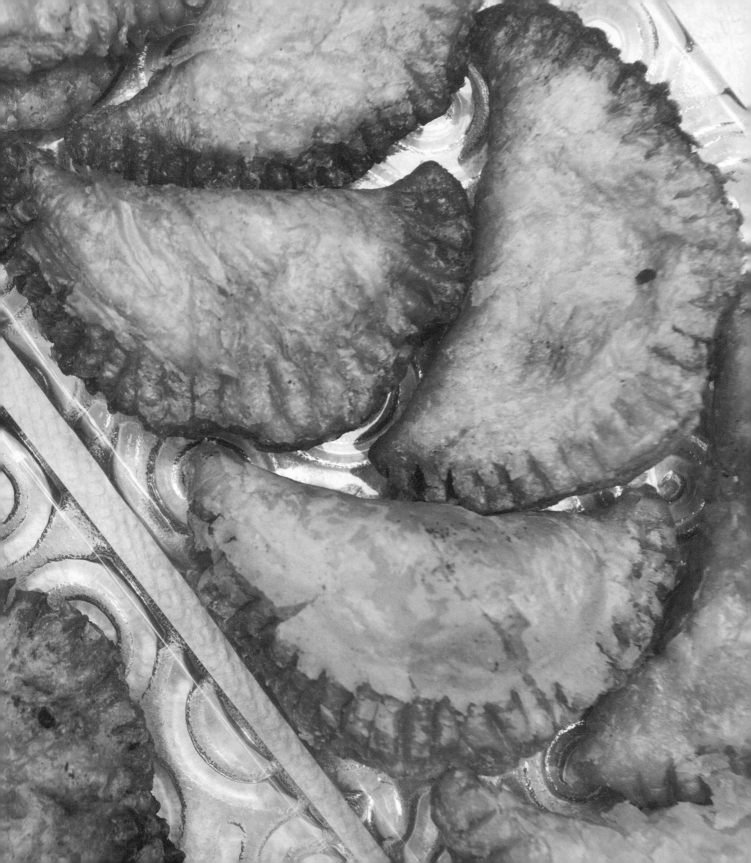

Crab and Cheese Empanadas

Empanadas are the Hispanic category of small pastry turnovers, and these are quite delicate. The filling joins morsels of prized crabmeat with Monterey Jack, a subtle cheese.

Yield: 2 dozen

Active time: 20 minutes

Start to finish: 55 minutes

2 tablespoons olive oil

2 large shallots, chopped

3 garlic cloves, minced

1 jalapeño or serrano chile, seeds and ribs removed, and chopped

¾ pound lump crabmeat, picked over well

¾ cup grated Monterey Jack

3 tablespoons chopped fresh cilantro

¼ teaspoon dried oregano, preferably Mexican

Salt and freshly ground black pepper to taste

1 batch Empanada Dough (page 130)

1 large egg, lightly beaten

1. Preheat the oven to 375°F. Cover two baking sheets with heavy-duty aluminum foil, and grease the foil.

2. Heat oil in a skillet over medium-high heat. Add shallots, garlic, and chile. Cook, stirring frequently, for 3 minutes, or until shallots are translucent. Remove the pan from the heat, and stir in crabmeat, cheese, cilantro, and oregano. Season to taste with salt and pepper. Allow mixture to cool.

3. Coat your rolling pin and your counter or mat with rice flour. Roll dough to ⅛-inch. Cut out 12 rounds using a 4-inch round biscuit cutter, reroll scraps as necessary. Repeat with remaining dough. Combine egg and 3 tablespoons water, and mix well.

4. Spoon 2 tablespoons filling onto one side of each pastry circle, leaving a ½-inch border. Brush edges with egg wash, and fold dough over filling to form a semicircle. Seal edges by pressing them together with the tines of a fork.

5. Place empanadas on baking sheets, and brush the tops with additional egg wash. Prick tops with the tines of a fork to allow steam to escape. Bake for 30 minutes, until the pastry is golden brown.

Note: The empanadas can be prepared for baking up to 1 day in advance and refrigerated, tightly covered. They can also be baked up to 3 days in advance. Reheat them in a 350°F oven for 7–10 minutes, or until hot.

Variations:
* *Substitute jalapeño Jack for the Monterey Jack for a spicier filling.*
* *Substitute shrimp or lobster for the crabmeat.*

Pre-picked-over crab meat from the seafood department is a tremendous time-saver, but it's far from perfect. The best way to ensure that no shell fragments find their way into a dish is to spread out the crab on a dark-colored plate. You'll see many fragments against the dark background so you can pick them out easily. Then rub the morsels between your fingers, being careful not to break up large lumps.

Beef Empanadas

The filling for these crispy turnovers is similar to traditional Mexican picadillo. *It's a variation on chili, with olives and raisins providing some sweet and sour nuances.*

Yield: 2 dozen

Active time: 20 minutes

Start to finish: 55 minutes

2 tablespoons olive oil, divided

¾ **pound lean ground beef**

1 medium onion, diced

3 garlic cloves, minced

1 tablespoon chili powder

1 tablespoon smoked Spanish paprika (*pimentón de la vera*)

1 teaspoon ground cumin

1 (8-ounce) can tomato sauce

¼ cup chopped pimiento-stuffed green olives

¼ cup chopped raisins

Salt and freshly ground black pepper to taste

1 batch Empanada Dough (page 130)

1 large egg, lightly beaten

1. Heat 1 tablespoon oil in a skillet over medium-high heat. Crumble beef into the skillet and brown well. Remove beef from the skillet with a slotted spoon, and set aside. Discard fat from the skillet.

2. Heat remaining oil in the skillet. Add onion and garlic, and cook, stirring frequently, for 3 minutes, or until onion is translucent. Stir in chili powder, paprika, and cumin. Cook for 1 minute, stirring constantly.

3. Return beef to the pan, and add tomato sauce, olives, and raisins. Bring to a boil, then reduce the heat to low and simmer for 15 minutes, or until thickened and beef is tender. Season to taste with salt and pepper. Allow filling to cool.

4. Preheat the oven to 375°F. Cover two baking sheets with heavy-duty aluminum foil, and grease the foil.

5. Coat your rolling pin and your counter or mat with rice flour. Roll dough to ⅛-inch. Cut out 12 rounds using a 4-inch round biscuit cutter, reroll scraps as necessary. Repeat with remaining dough. Combine egg and 3 tablespoons water, and mix well.

6. Spoon 2 tablespoons filling onto one side of each pastry circle, leaving a ½-inch border. Brush edges with egg wash, and fold dough over filling to form a semicircle. Seal edges by pressing them together with the tines of a fork.

7. Place empanadas on baking sheets, and brush the tops with additional egg wash. Prick tops with the tines of a fork to allow steam to escape. Bake for 30 minutes, until the pastry is golden brown.

Note: The empanadas can be prepared for baking up to 1 day in advance and refrigerated, tightly covered. They can also be baked up to 3 days in advance. Reheat them in a 350°F oven for 7–10 minutes, or until hot.

Variations:
* *Substitute Mexico chorizo, ground turkey, or ground pork for the beef.*
* *Add 2 chipotle chiles in adobo sauce, finely chopped, to the filling for a spicier dish.*

The purpose of an egg wash is to give pastry a browned and shiny crust. But it's important to brush the crust before cutting the steam vents because the egg wash can clog the vents, which will create a soggy crust.

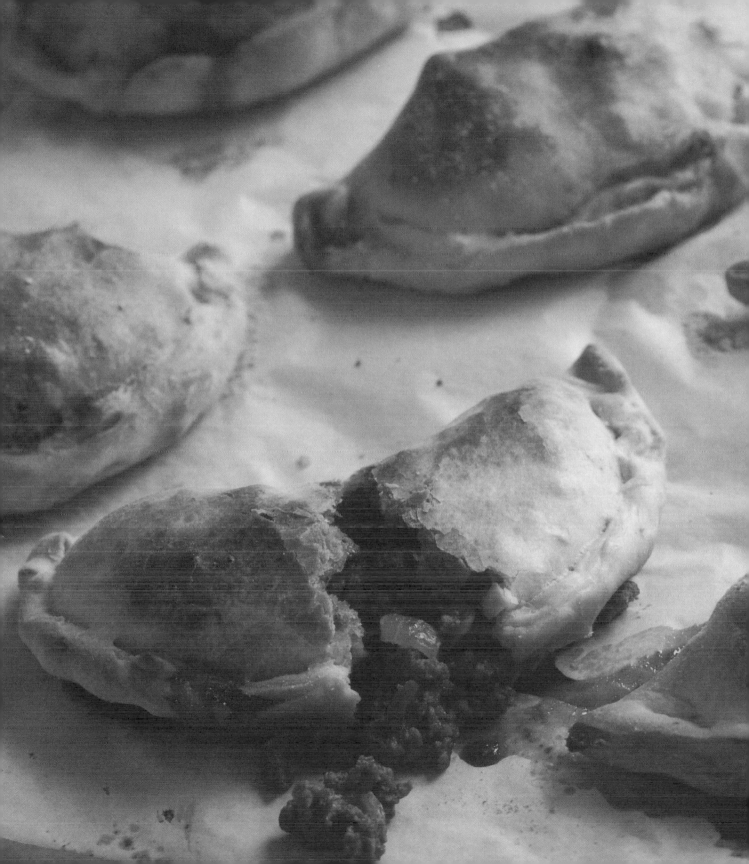

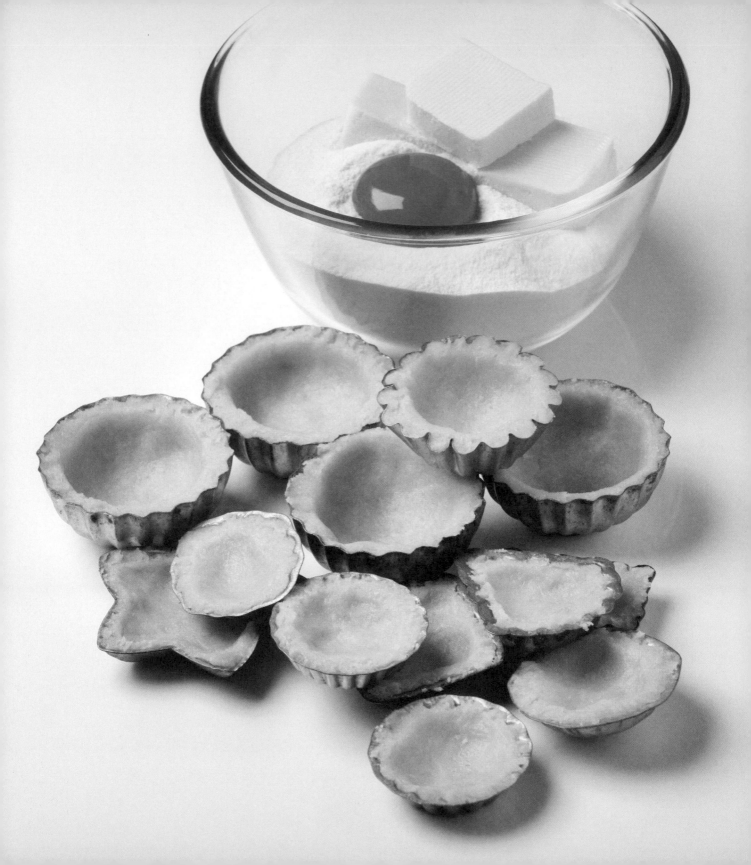

Basic Tartlet Crust

With a batch of this easy-to-make dough in the freezer you can create a huge range of fancy and delicious tartlets in merely minutes. Convert any of your favorite quiche recipes, or just bake the shells and fill them with a soft cheese.

Yield: enough for 2 dozen tartlets

Active time: 15 minutes

Start to finish: 15 minutes

2 cups brown rice flour

1½ cups potato starch

½ cup tapioca flour

1 teaspoon xanthan gum

½ teaspoon salt

¾ cup (1½ sticks) unsalted butter, chilled

2 large eggs

⅓ cup ice water

1. Combine brown rice flour, potato starch, tapioca flour, xanthan gum, and salt in a mixing bowl, and whisk well. Cut butter into cubes the size of lima beans, and cut into dry ingredients using a pastry blender, two knives, or your fingertips until mixture forms pea-sized chunks. This can also be done in a food processor fitted with the steel blade using on-and-off pulsing.

2. Combine eggs with ice water in a small bowl, and whisk well. Sprinkle mixture over dough, 1 tablespoon at a time. Toss lightly with fork until dough forms a ball. If using a food processor, process until mixture holds together when pressed between two fingers.

3. Divide dough in half, and form into a flat "pancake." Wrap each "pancake" in plastic wrap, and chill for at least 30 minutes. Roll and fill dough per instructions in individual recipes.

Note: The crust can be prepared up to 3 days in advance and refrigerated, tightly covered. Also, both dough "pancakes" and rolled out sheets can be frozen for up to 3 months.

> **Improvisation is the name of the game when it comes to kitchen equipment. No fancy round cutters in your kitchen? No problem. Look for a drinking glass, cup, or even a metal can in the recycling bin with the correct diameter and you're all set. Don't have a rolling pin? Cover a glass bottle with aluminum foil and use it to roll dough.**

Herbed Sausage and Tomato Tartlets

Yield: 2 dozen

Active time: 25 minutes

Start to finish: 40 minutes

1 batch Basic Tartlet Crust
(page 137)

¾ pound bulk sage pork
sausage

3 garlic cloves, minced

2 shallots, minced

4 ripe plum tomatoes, cored,
seeded, and finely chopped

1 tablespoon herbes
de Provence

Pinch of crushed
red pepper flakes

3 large eggs

1 cup heavy cream

Salt and freshly ground
black pepper to taste

1. Break off 2-teaspoons pieces of dough and press them evenly into the prepared cups, making the bottoms slightly thinner than the sides. Refrigerate for 30 minutes, or until dough firms again.

2. Preheat the oven to 375°F. Grease the cups in 2 (12-cup) mini-muffin pans.

3. Prick bottom and sides of cups with the tines of a fork. Bake for 8–10 minutes, or until set. Set aside.

4. Place a skillet over medium heat and crumble sausage into it, breaking up any lumps with a fork. Cook sausage, stirring occasionally, for 5 minutes, or until sausage is brown with no pink remaining. Add garlic and shallots and cook for 2 minutes. Add tomatoes and herbes de Provence, and red pepper flakes, and cook for 5–7 minutes, or until juice has evaporated. Cool mixture for 10 minutes.

5. Whisk eggs with cream and stir in cooled sausage mixture. Season to taste with salt and pepper. Spoon mixture into partially baked tartlet cups. Bake for 12–14 minutes, or until browned. Serve immediately.

Note: The sausage mixture can be prepared 1 day in advance and refrigerated, tightly covered. It does not need to be reheated, but do add 5 minutes to the baking time.

Variation:
∗ *Substitute Italian sausage for the sage sausage, Italian seasoning for the herbes de Provence, and add 3 tablespoons freshly grated Parmesan cheese to the filling.*

> *Pinch* is a term used for the amount of a dry ingredient that can be held between the tips of the thumb and forefinger of one hand. The smallest standard measuring spoon is ¼ teaspoon; a pinch is far less.

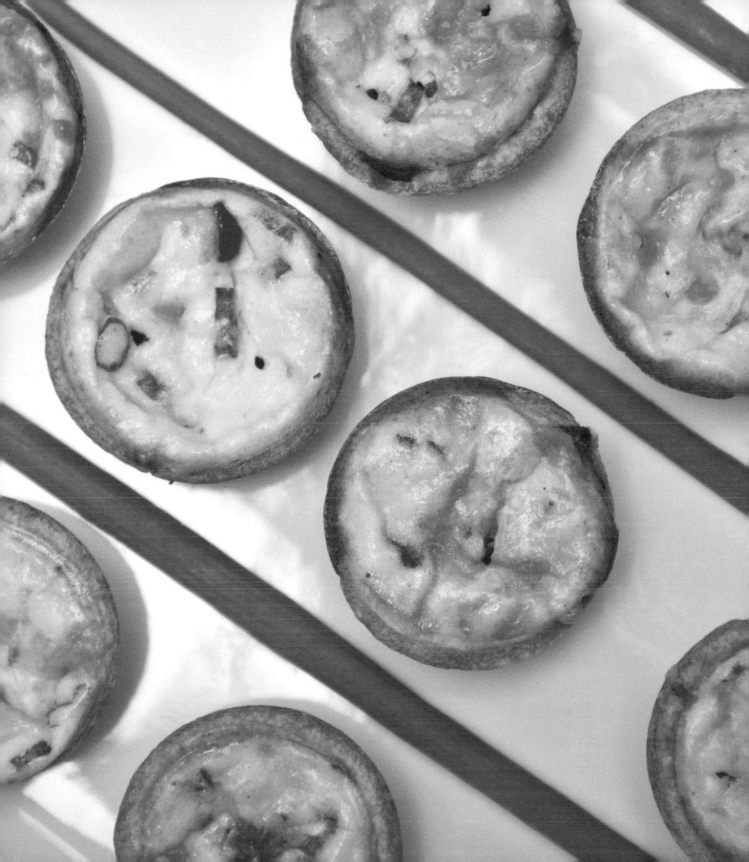

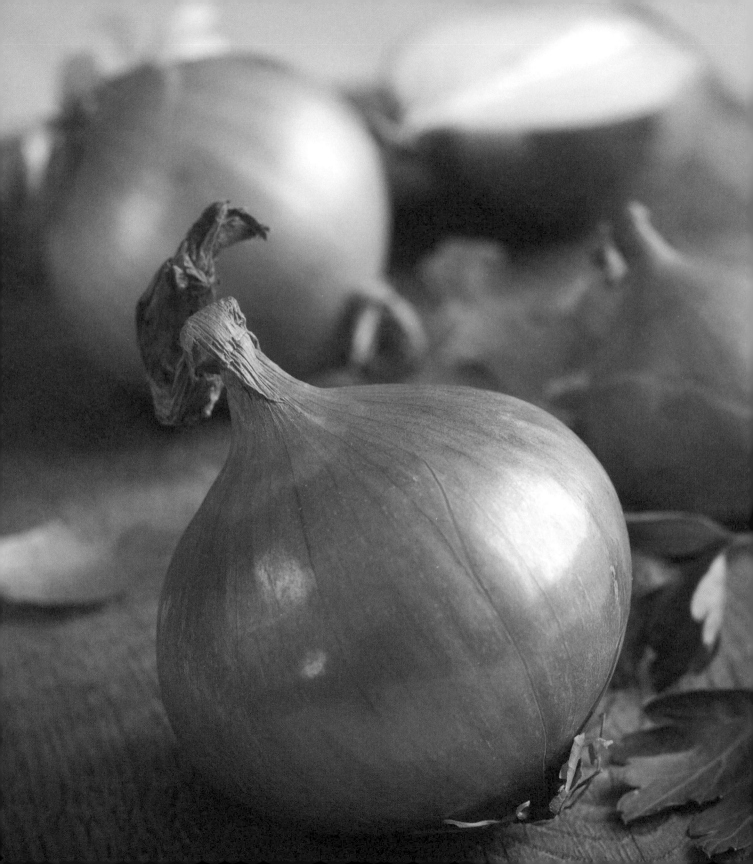

Caramelized Onion Tarts

If I had to choose a favorite vegetable ingredient it would be sweet caramelized onions. I love onion soup; I add the onions to mashed potatoes; and I use them to flavor this easy-to-prepare quiche.

Yield: 2 dozen

Active time: 30 minutes

Start to finish: 45 minutes

2 tablespoons unsalted butter

1 tablespoon olive oil

3 large onions, peeled and thinly sliced

Salt and freshly ground black pepper to taste

1 teaspoon granulated sugar

1 batch Basic Tartlet Dough (page 137)

3 large eggs

1 cup heavy cream

½ cup grated Gruyère or Swiss cheese

1. Heat butter and oil in a large skillet over low heat. Add onions, toss to coat, and cover the pan. Cook over low heat for 10 minutes, stirring occasionally. Uncover the pan, raise the heat to medium-high, sprinkle with salt and pepper, and stir in sugar. Cook for 25–30 minutes, stirring frequently, or until onions are dark brown. If the onions stick to the pan, stir to incorporate the browned juices into the onions. Cool the onions for 10 minutes.

2. While onions cook, break off 2-teaspoons pieces of dough and press them evenly into the prepared cups, making the bottoms slightly thinner than the sides. Refrigerate for 30 minutes, or until dough firms again.

3. Preheat the oven to 375°F. Grease the cups in 2 (12-cup) mini-muffin pans.

4. Prick bottom and sides of cups with the tines of a fork. Bake for 8–10 minutes, or until set. Set aside.

5. Whisk eggs with cream and stir in cheese and cooled onions. Season to taste with salt and pepper. Spoon mixture into partially baked tartlet cups. Bake for 12–14 minutes, or until browned. Serve immediately.

Note: The onions can be prepared 2 days in advance and refrigerated, tightly covered. They do not need to be reheated, but do add 5 minutes to the baking time.

Variations:
* *Substitute sharp Cheddar or smoked Cheddar for the Gruyère.*
* *Add 3 tablespoons finely chopped prosciutto or crumbled crisp bacon to the filling.*

> Onions are much easier to slice and dice if you start by cutting them in half through the root end. That way the halves sit firmly on your cutting board.

INDEX

About the Author

Ellen Brown is a well-respected author of more than thirty cookbooks.

These include the following titles from Cider Mill Press: *The Meatball Cookbook Bible*, *The Sausage Cookbook Bible*, *Gluten-Free Slow Cooking*, and *Italian Slow Cooking*. *Very Vegan Christmas Cookies* will also be published in 2012.

As the founding food writer of *USA Today*, Ellen gained the national spotlight in 1982. Since then, Ellen's writing has appeared in dozens of publications, including the *Washington Post, Bon Appetit*, and *Good Food Dossier*.

Ellen lives in Providence, Rhode Island and writes a weekly column for *The Providence Journal*, featuring a variety of original recipes.

About Appleseed Press Book Publishers

Great ideas grow over time. From seed to harvest, Appleseed Press
brings fine reading and entertainment together between the covers
of its creatively crafted books. Our grove bears fruit twice a year,
publishing a new crop of titles each Spring and Fall.

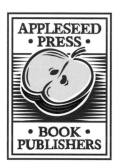

Visit us on the Web at
www.appleseedpressbooks.com
or write to us at
68 North Street
Kennebunkport, Maine 04046